WHO Technical Report Series

Research Priorities for Helminth Infections

Technical Report of the TDR Disease Reference Group on Helminth Infections

This report contains the collective views of an international group of experts and does not necessarily represent the decisions or the stated policy of the World Health Organization

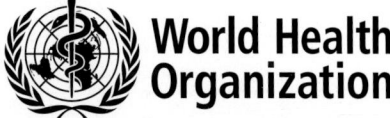

WHO Library Cataloguing-in-Publication Data

Research priorities for helminth infections: technical report of the TDR disease reference group on helminth infections.

(Technical report series ; no. 972)

1. Helminthiasis - prevention and control. 2. Research. 3. Neglected diseases. 4. Poverty. I.World Health Organization. II.Series.

ISBN 978 92 4 120972 4   (NLM classification: WC 800)
ISSN 0512-3054

© World Health Organization 2012

All rights reserved. Publications of the World Health Organization are available on the WHO web site (www.who.int) or can be purchased from WHO Press, World Health Organization, 20 Avenue Appia, 1211 Geneva 27, Switzerland (tel.: +41 22 791 3264; fax: +41 22 791 4857; e-mail: bookorders@who.int).

Requests for permission to reproduce or translate WHO publications – whether for sale or for noncommercial distribution – should be addressed to WHO Press through the WHO web site (http://www.who.int/about/licensing/copyright_form/en/index.html).

The designations employed and the presentation of the material in this publication do not imply the expression of any opinion whatsoever on the part of the World Health Organization concerning the legal status of any country, territory, city or area or of its authorities, or concerning the delimitation of its frontiers or boundaries. Dotted lines on maps represent approximate border lines for which there may not yet be full agreement.

The mention of specific companies or of certain manufacturers' products does not imply that they are endorsed or recommended by the World Health Organization in preference to others of a similar nature that are not mentioned. Errors and omissions excepted, the names of proprietary products are distinguished by initial capital letters.

All reasonable precautions have been taken by the World Health Organization to verify the information contained in this publication. However, the published material is being distributed without warranty of any kind, either expressed or implied. The responsibility for the interpretation and use of the material lies with the reader. In no event shall the World Health Organization be liable for damages arising from its use.

This publication contains the collective views of an international group of experts and does not necessarily represent the decisions or the policies of the World Health Organization.

Printed in Italy

Contents

The TDR Disease Reference Group on Helminth Infections	vii
Acronyms and abbreviations	ix
List of species	xiii
Executive summary	xv

1. Introduction   1
- 1.1 The problem of helminthiases   1
- 1.2 Human helminthiases, populations at risk and resulting diseases   6
- 1.3 Group membership   12
- 1.4 Host country   14
- 1.5 Think Tank members   14

2. Methodology and prioritization   15
- 2.1 Identification of the helminth infections to be considered   15
- 2.2 Identification of the research gaps to be considered   16
- 2.3 The first DRG4 meeting   17
- 2.4 Prioritization of themes   19
  - 2.4.1 Underlying values   19
  - 2.4.2 Criteria for ranking   19
- 2.5 The second DRG4 meeting   20
- 2.6 Ranking of priority research areas by experts in DRG4   20
- 2.7 Stakeholders consultation meetings and other external contributions   21
  - 2.7.1 First stakeholders' consultation   21
  - 2.7.2 Second stakeholders' consultation   21
- 2.8 Publication of the DRG4 report   22

3. Overview of trends and driving forces of persistent, emerging and re-emerging helminth infections and the consequent research and control challenges   23
- 3.1 Parasite population biology and human host sociological factors   23
- 3.2 Chemotherapeutic factors   24
- 3.3 Factors associated with current ability to diagnose helminth infections in individuals, communities and larger spatial scales   25
- 3.4 Factors associated with the environmental and social ecology of human helminthiases   27
- 3.5 Factors associated with research gaps in basic helminth biology   28

4. Overview of significant recent advances for the control and elimination of helminth infections and deeper analysis of control challenges and research issues for helminth diseases   31
- 4.1 Advances in interventions and their monitoring and evaluation   31
- 4.2 Analysis of the tools for control interventions   34
  - 4.2.1 Anthelmintic pharmaceuticals and their modalities of delivery   34
  - 4.2.2 Efficacy of anthelmintics   40
  - 4.2.3 Anthelmintic resistance   40

		4.2.4	Combinations of anthelmintics	44
		4.2.5	Vector control	46
		4.2.6	Vaccines	47
	4.3	Advances in tools for diagnosis of infection and surveillance of interventions		48
	4.4	Analysis of the tools for diagnosis, monitoring and evaluation, and surveillance and their challenges		48
		4.4.1	Diagnostics for filariases	52
		4.4.2	Diagnostics for soil-transmitted helminthiases	57
		4.4.3	Diagnostics for schistosomiasis (including infections by *Schistosoma mansoni*, *S. haematobium* and *S. japonicum*)	60
		4.4.4	Diagnostics for taeniasis (*Taenia solium*/cysticercosis)	63
	4.5	Issues related to bringing new diagnostics to market		65
	4.6	Advances in mathematical modelling of helminth infections		67
	4.7	Advances in the understanding of pathology and assessment of morbidity		68
	4.8	Analysis of the challenges for epidemiological data and mathematical models		72
		4.8.1	Transmission thresholds	72
		4.8.2	Parasite population biology factors	72
		4.8.3	Co-infections, multiple populations, and niche-shifts	74
		4.8.4	Infection and disease mapping	74
		4.8.5	Morbidity control vs. elimination	74
		4.8.6	Transition from endemic to post-control parasite biology and ecology	75
	4.9	Advances in helminth biology		76
		4.9.1	Parasite genomics and functional genomics	76
		4.9.2	Transmission biology	79
		4.9.3	Immunology	79
		4.9.4	Host-parasite interaction and pathology	81
		4.9.5	Vector-filaria and snail-schistosome interactions	83
	4.10	Analysis of challenges stemming from gaps in knowledge of basic helminth biology		85
		4.10.1	Host-parasite interaction and immunopathology	85
		4.10.2	Other aspects of basic biology	89
		4.10.3	Vector-filaria and snail-trematode interactions	92

5. Intersectoral and cross-cutting issues 95

	5.1	Cross-cutting issues of participation, ownership, empowerment, equity and gender	95
	5.2	The impact of global climate change	96
	5.3	Challenges stemming from environmental and social ecology factors: water-associated diseases and water management	97
	5.4	Limitations in the health services	97
	5.5	Polyparasitism and integration of intervention measures	98

6. Regional highlights and research capacity 101

	6.1	Regional highlights		101
	6.2	Research capacity		102
		6.2.1	Background	102
		6.2.2	Inequalities in research capacity	103
		6.2.3	Research capacity in disease-endemic countries	104
		6.2.4	Challenges for research capacity building in disease-endemic countries	107
		6.2.5	National, regional, and global efforts and strategies towards capacity building for research in infectious diseases of poverty	111

7. Regional and national policies on research and their implications   115
    7.1   Background   115
    7.2   Regional health research policies   115
    7.3   National health research policies   116
    7.4   Recommendations   117

8. Research priority recommendations to policy and decision-makers   119
    8.1   Intervention   120
    8.2   Epidemiology and surveillance   120
    8.3   Environment and social ecology   121
    8.4   Data and modelling   121
    8.5   Biology research   122

9. Conclusions   123

Acknowledgements   125

References   127

Annex 1
The TDR disease and thematic reference groups Think Tank for Infectious Diseases of Poverty, and host countries   155

Annex 2
Membership of the Disease Reference Group on Helminth Infections (DRG4)   157

Annex 3
Composition of the Think Tank   159

Annex 4
Distribution of the Think Tank leadership (co-Chairs)   167

Annex 5
The top ten research priority areas for helminthiases recommended by DRG4   169

Annex 6
Research landmarks and their projected impacts on the helminthiases in the short, mid and long-term periods   173

WHO/TDR Disease Reference Group on Helminth Infections (DRG4) 2009-2010

Members

Dr K. Awadzi, Director, Onchocerciasis Chemotherapy Research Centre, Hohoe, Ghana*

Dr R.M. Barakat, Professor, Medical Parasitology, High Institute of Public Health, Alexandria University, Alexandria, Egypt

Professor M.G. Basáñez, Chair in Neglected Tropical Diseases, and Head, Helminth Ecology Research Group, Department of Infectious Disease Epidemiology, School of Public Health, Faculty of Medicine (St Mary's Campus), Imperial College London, England

Dr B. Boatin, Adjunct Professor, Institute of Parasitology, McGill University, Montreal, Canada, and Chief Scientific Advisor, Lymphatic Filariasis Support Centre, Department of Parasitology, Noguchi Memorial Institute for Medical Research, University of Ghana, Accra, Ghana (*Co-Chair*)

Professor H.H. García, Department of Microbiology, and Director of the Center for Global Health - Tumbes, Universidad Peruana Cayetano Heredia, Lima, Peru; and Head, Cysticercosis Unit, Instituto de Ciencias Neurológicas, Lima, Peru

Dr A. Gazzinelli, Professor, School of Nursing, Federal University of Minas Gerais, Brazil

Dr W. Grant, Associate Professor, Reader and Head, Genetic Department, La Trobe University, Bundoora, Australia

Dr S. Lustigman, Member and Head, Laboratory of Molecular Parasitology, Lindsley F. Kimball Research Institute, USA (*Chair*)

Professor J. McCarthy, Clinical Tropical Medicine Laboratory, Queensland Institute of Medical Research, University of Queensland, Herston' QLD, Australia

Professor K.E. N'Goran, Laboratoire de Zoologie et de Biologie Animale, Université de Cocody, Abidjan, Côte d'Ivoire

Professor R.K. Prichard, James McGill Professor, Institute of Parasitology, McGill University, Quebec, Canada

Professor B. Sripa, Head, Tropical Disease Research Laboratory, Faculty of Medicine, Khon Kaen University, Thailand

Professor G.J. Yang, Vice Head of Department Schistosomiasis Control, Jiangsu Institute of Parasitic Diseases, Wuxi, China

---

* Deceased, April 2011.

Career Development Fellow

Dr M.Y. Osei-Atweneboana, Senior Research Scientist, Laboratory of Medical Parasitology and Molecular Epidemiology, Council for Scientific and Industrial Research (CSIR), Department of Environmental Biology and Health, Water Research Institute, Accra, Ghana

Secretariat

Dr D. Kioy, Scientist, Special Programme for Research and Training in Tropical Diseases, World Health Organization, Geneva, Switzerland (*Secretary*)

Dr A.M.J Oduola, Coordinator, Special Programme for Research and Training in Tropical Diseases, World Health Organization, Geneva, Switzerland

Dr A.L. Willingham, Scientist, Special Programme for Research and Training in Tropical Diseases, World Health Organization, Geneva, Switzerland

Dr M. Wilson, Scientist, Special Programme for Research and Training in Tropical Diseases, World Health Organization, Geneva, Switzerland

Acronyms and abbreviations

Abs	Antibodies
ABC-transporters	ATP binding cassette transporters
ABZ	Albendazole
ADLA	Acute dermatolymphangioadenitis
ANDI	African Network for Drugs and Diagnostics Innovation
APOC	African Programme for Onchocerciasis Control
APOD	Acute papular onchodermatitis
ATR	Atrophy of the skin in onchocerciasis
BioMalPar	Biology and pathology of malaria parasite
BLAST	Basic local alignment search tool
BZ	Benzimidazole
CAA	Circulating anodic antigen
CCA	Circulating cathodic antigen
CFA	Circulating filarial antigen
ComDT	Community-directed treatment
CDTI	Community-directed treatment with ivermectin
CPOD	Chronic papular onchodermatitis
DALY	Disability-adjusted life-year
DEC	Diethylcarbamazine
DFID	Department for International Development (UK)
DPM	Depigmentation of the skin in onchocerciasis
DRG	Disease Reference Group
DtW	Deworm the World
ECP	Eosinophil cationic protein
ELISA	Enzyme-linked immunosorbent assay
Epg	Eggs per gram of faeces
ES	Excretory-secretory

ERR	Egg reduction rate	
EST	Expressed sequence tag	
FDA	Food and Drug Administration (USA)	
FERCT	Faecal egg reduction count test	
FIND	Foundation for Innovative New Diagnostics	
GIS	Geographic information system	
GNNTDC	Global Network for Neglected Tropical Disease Control	
GPELF	Global Programme to Eliminate Lymphatic filariasis	
GDP	Gross domestic product	
HG	Hanging groin in onchocerciasis	
ICT	Immunochromatographic card test	
IHA	Indirect haemagglutination assay	
IL	Interleukin	
IVM	Ivermectin	
JICA	Japanese International Cooperation Agency	
KK	Kato Katz test	
LANBIO	Latin American Network for Research on Bioactive Natural Compounds	
LE	Lymphoedema	
LEC	Lymphatic endothelial cells	
LF	Lymphatic filariasis	
LaoPDR	Lao People's Democratic Republic	
LOD	Lichenified onchodermatitis	
LYM	Lymphatic involvement in onchocerciasis	
mf	Microfilariae	
MBZ	Mebendazole	
MDA	Mass drug administration	
MDG	Millennium development goal	
MDSS	Medical Device Safety Service of the European Union	
M&E	Monitoring and evaluation	

MICT	Magnetic immunochromatographic card test
MSAT	Mass screen and treat
NCC	Neurocysticercosis
NEPAD	New Partnership for Africa's Development
NTD	Neglected tropical disease
OAU	Organization of African Unity
OCP	Onchocerciasis Control Programme in West Africa
OEPA	Onchocerciasis Elimination Program for the Americas
OSD	Onchocercal skin disease
PAHO	Pan American Health Organization
PDIP	Product Development and Implementation Partnership
PBMC	Peripheral blood mononuclear cells
PCR	Polymerase chain reaction
PPC	Partners for Parasite Control
PZQ	Praziquantel
PRC	People's Republic of China
REA	Rapid epidemiological assessment
REMO	Rapid epidemiological mapping of onchocerciasis
RNAi	RNA interference
RS	Remote sensing
SAE	Severe adverse events
SEA	Soluble egg antigen
SCI	Schistosomiasis Control Initiative
SNP	Single nucleotide polymorphism
SSA	Sub-Saharan Africa
STH	Soil-transmitted helminthiasis
TDR	UNICEF/UNDP/World Bank/WHO Special Programme for Research and Training in Tropical Diseases
Th	T helper cell
TLR	Toll-like receptor

TNF	Tumor necrosis factor	
TRG	Thematic reference group	
VEGF	Vascular endothelial growth factors	
WHA	World Health Assembly	
WHO	World Health Organization	
WSP	*Wolbachia* surface protein	

List of species

Aedes spp.
Ascaris lumbricoides
Ancylostoma duodenale
Ancylostoma caninum
Ancylostoma ceylanicum
Anopheles spp.
Biomphalaria glabrata
Brugia malayi
Brugia timori
Bulinus globosus
Clonorchis sinensis
Culex quinquefasciatus
Echinococcus multilocularis
Fasciola hepatica
Fasciolopsis buski
Helicobacter pylori
Loa loa
Necator americanus
Ochlerotatus niveus
Onchocerca volvulus
Onchocerca ochengi
Oncomelania hupensis
Opisthorchis felineus
Opisthorchis viverrini
Paragonimus spp.
Plasmodium spp.
Schistosoma bovis
Schistosoma haematobium
Schistosoma japonicum
Schistosoma mansoni
Simulium damnosum
Simulium neavei
Simulium yahense
Strongyloides stercoralis
Taenia crassiceps
Taenia saginata
Taenia solium
Trichuris trichiura
Wolbachia spp.
Wuchereria bancrofti

Executive summary

The Disease Reference Group on Helminth Infections (DRG4) is part of an independent think tank of international experts, established by TDR, the Special Programme for Research and Training in Tropical Diseases, to identify key research priorities. The mandate of DRG4 was to evaluate information on research and challenges in helminthiases of public health importance, including onchocerciasis, lymphatic filariasis, soil-transmitted helminthiases, schistosomiasis, food-borne trematodiases and taeniasis/cysticercosis.

This report summarizes, in a comprehensive and integrated fashion, current helminth research issues and opportunities for improving disease control and reducing poverty. It identifies research gaps and challenges, and presents recommendations to inform public health policy, guide implementation programmes, and focus the research community on the dire needs and the opportunities for advancing disease control and improving human welfare.

Helminthiases affect human populations particularly in marginalized, resource-constrained regions of the world. Over one billion people in sub-Saharan Africa, Asia and the Americas are infected with one or more helminth species. The morbidity from such infections maintains a vicious circle of poverty, decreased productivity, and inadequate socioeconomic development. Furthermore, helminth infection can exacerbate malaria and HIV/AIDS, and impair vaccine efficacy. Polyparasitism is common and infections tend to be long lasting and stable. Major deficiencies exist in current control tools, diagnostics, and fundamental knowledge of helminth biology and transmission dynamics. Despite some promising leads for the development of anti-helminth vaccines e.g. the TSOL18 porcine vaccine for cysticercosis, there is a dearth of vaccines for human helminthiases. Adequate diagnostics and surveillance are crucial for sustained helminth control. Among the challenges for surveillance and evaluation are: quantification of infection intensity and of response to anthelmintic, including detection of drug resistance, and determination of transmission end-points.

Therefore, there is a need for: 1) updated disease prevalence maps; 2) more sensitive diagnostics; 3) monitoring the progress of control interventions and quantifying changes in incidence of infection and disease; 4) assessing drug efficacy and promptly detecting development of drug resistance; 5) determining programme end-points (for elimination of infection); 6) post-control surveillance; and 7) developing appropriate health research policies and capacity building in disease-endemic countries to provide conducive environment and adequate expertise for sustained disease control efforts.

There have been demonstrated successes and an expansion of tools. These include: making affordable safe anthelmintics which can be delivered through mass drug administration, advances in epidemiological mapping, monitoring and evaluation protocols, tools for infection diagnosis and surveillance, understanding the pathogenesis of infections and the relationship between infection and disease burden, mathematical models for transmission dynamics and control, antiparasitic vaccines, and parasite genomics. Geographical information systems and remote sensing have aided epidemiology and disease mapping. Furthermore, some research capacity has been developed in disease-endemic countries through North–South collaborations.

However, analysis of the information shows that further research is needed to address control challenges. While most helminth control programmes concentrate heavily on treatment, with positive results, they do not incorporate environmental considerations and health education that can facilitate programme integration and sustainability. Research is needed to optimize control strategies, quantify their cost–effectiveness, and establish how these strategies impact infection, morbidity, and compliance. Additionally, the paucity of pharmaceuticals for elimination is of concern in view of increasing mass drug administration in large-scale programmes and the real possibility of drug resistance. Crucially, political will and commitment, and investing in South–South collaborations, will be pivotal for developing appropriate research policies and capacity in disease-endemic countries, as well as for implementing the research and development agenda in controlling and eliminating the human helminthiases discussed here.

Five major core themes were identified as umbrella priorities, namely, intervention, epidemiology and surveillance, environmental and social ecology, data and modelling, and fundamental biology. Amongst these themes, ten priority research areas were identified (Box 1). For effective control of helminthiasis, in addition to the five core research themes, there is also the need for appropriate health research policies and research capacity building in disease-endemic countries. The recommendations are grounded on the notion that research is needed in order to improve and update our knowledge of helminth infections and in order to translate such knowledge into intervention tools. Finally, it is imperative that across the spectrum, from village level to the highest international level, better understanding and appreciation be promoted of the importance of human helminthiases as causes of ill-health and extreme poverty, so that resources for combating such infections may be greatly increased.

Executive summary

Box 1
The top ten priority research areas for helminth infections

1. Research to optimize existing intervention tools to maximize impact and sustainability (including tools against polyparasitism). The tools include pharmaceuticals, vaccines, vector control and ecohealth approaches (including improvements in sanitation, access to clean water, nutrition, and education). Sustainability depends on maintaining community support and minimizing selection for drug resistance.
2. Research to develop novel control tools to improve impact and sustainability. The tools include pharmaceuticals, vaccines, vector control and ecohealth approaches, and how to deliver them optimally and cost effectively.
3. Research to improve available diagnostic tests, specifically their sensitivity, specificity, multiplex capacity, and ability to measure infection intensity, and detect drug resistance. Sensitivity and specificity are crucially important to enable diagnosis of infection at low prevalence, in elimination settings, and to confirm cure/absence of infection.
4. Research to standardize and validate methodologies and cost-effective protocols for diagnosis in the process of monitoring and evaluation (M&E).
5. Research to develop strategies incorporating delivery of multiple interventions at various levels to maximize sustainability of control programmes in general, and of integrated neglected tropical diseases (NTD) control in particular.
6. Research to develop strategies (taking gender issues into account) to increase: awareness of ill-health processes, community participation, ownership and empowerment, as well as equity in access to health services for communities and risk groups.
7. Research to develop and refine mathematical models to investigate relationships between infection and morbidities to aid programmes aiming to reduce the burden of disease (elimination of public health problem). Such models need to take into account cumulative effects of chronic disease for evaluation of disease burden and the impact on such burden of control interventions.
8. Research to increase use and application of epidemiological models to aid M&E and surveillance, the design of cost-effective sampling protocols and the monitoring of intervention efficacy including drug resistance. These models should be linked to cost-effectiveness analyses of the interventions and their alternatives.
9. Research how helminth parasites modulate host–parasite interactions at the population and within-host levels, including the impact on the host immune response of concurrent infection with other helminth and non-helminth pathogens, the impact of parasite control interventions on such host–parasite interactions, and how concurrent infections affect clinical outcomes and the host's ability to seroconvert upon vaccination.
10. Research to annotate parasite genomes and transcriptomes, and to develop new tools for parasite functional genomics in key species.

1. Introduction

As part of a strategy[1] to foster "an effective global research effort on infectious diseases of poverty in which disease-endemic countries play a pivotal role", TDR established a global research Think Tank of 125 international experts to continually and systematically review evidence, assess research needs and, following periodic national and regional stakeholder consultations, to set research priorities for accelerating the control of infectious diseases of poverty. Working in ten disease-specific and thematic reference groups (DRGs/TRGs; see Annex 1), these experts have been crucial contributors to TDR's mandate for the acquisition and analysis of information on infectious diseases of poverty. Their work is intended to promote control-relevant research, achieve research innovation and to enhance the capacity of disease endemic countries to resolve public health problems related to the disproportionate burden of infectious diseases among the poor.

This report addresses the research needs for helminth infections and identifies research gaps and challenges, and presents research priorities for improving disease control. Research priorities identified by the Disease Reference group on Helminth Infections (DRG4) are presented and the methods used to reach these priorities are discussed.

1.1 The problem of helminthiases

Since the publication by Norman Stoll in 1947 of 'This Wormy World' (*1*), which raised awareness of the intolerable burden of intestinal nematode infections, several global efforts have been made to address the problem of human parasitism by helminths. Helminths (roundworm and flatworm parasites) are among the most widespread infectious agents that have affected, and still affect, human populations, particularly in marginalized, low-income and resource-constrained regions of the world. It is estimated that over one billion people in developing regions of sub-Saharan Africa (SSA), Asia and the Americas are infected with one or more species of helminths (*2, 3*). The morbidity associated with such infections imposes a substantial burden of disease, which helps establish and maintain a vicious circle of infection, poverty, decreased productivity, and inadequate socioeconomic development. The infections themselves may have an impact on other conditions such as malaria, HIV/AIDS, and the ability to respond effectively to a range of anti-infectious disease vaccines.

The increasing acknowledgement of the burden imposed by helminthiases, particularly since the last quarter of the 20th century, has led to the implementation of large-scale control and elimination programmes.

---

[1] Details of TDR's strategy can be found at http://www.who.int/tdr/about/

These were aimed at the parasites themselves and/or the agents (vectors and intermediate hosts) responsible for their transmission. In 1974, the World Health Assembly passed resolution WHA27.52 calling upon the World Health Organization (WHO) to intensify research on major parasitic diseases; this led to the creation of the Special Programme for Research and Training in Tropical Diseases (TDR) in 1975, which was sponsored by UNDP, the World Bank and WHO, and later, UNICEF. That year also saw the establishment of the Onchocerciasis Control Programme (OCP) in West Africa. In 1993 and 1995 respectively, the Onchocerciasis Elimination Program for the Americas (OEPA) and the African Programme for Onchocerciasis Control (APOC) were initiated. In 1997, the World Health Assembly (WHA) passed resolution WHA50.29, which urged the WHO and Member States to take advantage of recent advances and opportunities for lymphatic filariasis (LF) elimination, and led to the formation of the Global Alliance to Eliminate Lymphatic Filariasis (GPELF), consequently launched in 2000. In 2001, the WHA passed resolution WHA54.19, setting the global target of treating at least 75% of all school-aged children at risk of morbidity from soil-transmitted helminthiases (STHs) and schistosomiasis by the year 2010. This resolution led to the establishment of Partners for Parasite Control (PPC) by the WHO. More recently, the global public health community has had the fillip of the Millennium Development Goals (MDGs), and several new initiatives have been established, most notably the Schistosomiasis Control Initiative (SCI) in 2002, and the Global Network for Neglected Tropical Disease Control (GNNTDC) in 2006.

Most of the helminthic diseases on which this report focuses are closely linked to poverty; they result from poverty and markedly contribute to further poverty by, among other factors, impairing agricultural productivity, and effecting negative impacts on cognitive development and education (4, 5). In response to growing evidence that such neglected tropical diseases (NTDs) devastate the bottom billion of the world population through their effects on health, education, and socioeconomic development, the WHA has adopted several resolutions calling for the control or elimination of these diseases as described above.

Despite these resolutions and the many scientific advancements in our understanding of the biology and epidemiology of helminth infections, obstacles remain that challenge the global public health community. Identified obstacles include the scarcity of tools for: 1) updated disease mapping (particularly as interventions progress); 2) improved, more sensitive diagnostics that meet distinctive applications; 3) monitoring the progress of control interventions and quantifying changes in incidence of infection and disease; 4) assessing drug efficacy and promptly detecting possible development of drug resistance; 5) determining programme end-points (for elimination of the public health burden and/or the infection reservoir); and 6) implementing post-control surveillance.

Although the importance of ancillary strategies such as raising community recognition and ownership of the diseases present in the community and their associated problems, effecting environmental improvement, increasing hygiene practices and access to clean water, and sustaining socioeconomic development, is widely recognized, the mainstay of helminthiasis control has become the deployment of targeted treatment (to particular occupational or age groups), or of mass drug administration (MDA) to the wider community. The drugs (anthelmintics) involved are in some cases donated by pharmaceutical companies (e.g. ivermectin by Merck & Co. for onchocerciasis and LF, and albendazole by GlaxoSmithKline (GSK) for LF and STHs (6)), and in other cases are affordable as generic preparations (e.g. praziquantel for schistosomiasis, diethylcarbamazine for LF), making the MDA programmes among the most cost-effective global public health control measures. In general, the anthelmintic drugs adopted by the control programmes are safe for mass treatment of human populations and moderately to highly (albeit variably) effective.

MDA is being assisted by global partnerships, including the aforementioned donations of anthelmintic drugs by pharmaceutical companies, and donations of funds by foundations, governments, United Nations agencies, companies and individuals. Efforts to integrate various MDA programmes may bring logistic benefits to intervention efforts. However, it should also be recognized that very little funding is available to support the research that is necessary for interventions to remain sustainable and bring long-lasting benefits. Unfortunately, much of the effort is, at present, directed at short-term objectives.

Mass chemotherapy as a control strategy does indeed have its challenges, chiefly those of optimizing community involvement and participation. Recognition and acceptance by the community, and their commitment to play the role that is expected of them, also pose serious challenges to achieving sustainable control programmes. While global funding for the programmes has increased markedly in recent years, empathy tends to wane after the initial successes (which are invariably largest at the beginning), and 'donor fatigue' sets in as a major obstacle to sustained funding. Other issues include the fact that the arsenal of available drugs is limited – most of them were developed originally for parasites of veterinary importance in markets of middle to high income economies – and there is very little or no development of new drugs specifically targeted to human helminthiases. This makes the existing control programmes highly vulnerable should anthelmintic resistance develop and spread, as is theoretically likely with MDA programmes. Moreover, the long-term control and eradication of these helminth diseases will depend on increased sanitation and hygiene, improved socioeconomic development, and environmental sustainability.

The increasing size and activities of the human population, and the changing of agriculture and irrigation practices are also altering the environment at an unprecedented scale, further increasing the risk of zoonotic helminthiases as discussed in more detail in a separate report by the Disease Reference Group on Zoonoses and Marginalized Infectious Diseases of Poverty (DRG6). How these activities will play out in the long term, as well as what will be the effects of climate change on the distribution and incidence of helminth infections remains poorly understood. Thus, whereas helminth diseases are often thought of as chronic and ancient scourges of humanity, some may become re-emerging diseases as new outbreaks are reported in response to environmental and socio-political changes, migration, travel, forced human displacement, and clean water shortages.

Millions of doses of anthelmintics have been administered to patently infected and exposed individuals in endemic areas, in some cases for prolonged periods, and have undoubtedly yielded health benefits for the treated populations. However, helminth infections persist in their host populations and are resilient to control interventions (a consequence, in part, of their population biology). Understanding the biological, environmental and social determinants of such persistence, as well as the driving forces behind new emerging and re-emerging public health challenges is crucial to steering research, harnessing the potential of new scientific advancements, and engaging stakeholders to achieve the MDGs.

With all of the above influencing the success of human helminthiases control and elimination efforts, there is a clear need for an innovative research framework that is thoroughly integrated with the programmes, holistic in approach, collaborative and global in perspective, and that assesses current understanding, identifies gaps in knowledge, and seizes opportunities to address specific needs and move the helminth control agenda forward.

Reviews of progress in implementation of the MDGs indicate that attainment of the goals has been slow, particularly those related to health, namely MDG4 – reduce child mortality, MDG5 – improve maternal health, and MDG6 – combat HIV/AIDS, malaria and other diseases. This is particularly worrying for many African countries. This slow progress is not consistent with the actual increase in resources for health research worldwide; however, only 5% of global research spending is estimated to actually be applied to the needs of low and middle income countries and a miniscule fraction of this to the neglected helminth diseases. In fact, though MDG6 specifically mentions HIV/AIDS and malaria as critical targets for sustainable poverty reduction by the year 2015, it merely alludes to chronic parasitic worm infections as "other diseases" (2). Because these diseases prevent the achievement of the first six MDGs, their control with cost-effective interventions could be the basis for long-term economic growth and development (2).

Although the disability among the bottom billion that results from NTDs, including the helminth diseases, is enormous, the NTDs have not received nearly the same attention as three of the highest mortality-causing infectious diseases, HIV/AIDS, malaria, and tuberculosis (7), because they are not frequently perceived as major causes of premature death. However, onchocerciasis can cause visual impairment, blindness, and excess mortality both of the blind and of heavily infected yet sighted individuals; LF can cause major body deformation and impaired function, reducing the ability of people to work and look after themselves and others; STHs and schistosomiasis can markedly reduce the growth and development of children, including cognitive ability throughout life, as well as increase child mortality. Hookworm infection can cause anaemia and impact on maternal health and neonatal mortality; in pregnant women, the infections may result in premature birth, low birth weight and increased maternal morbidity and mortality. Liver fluke infections can cause major liver pathology, including hepatic cancer, while neurocysticercosis is a major cause of seizure disorders and other forms of neurological disease that can increase the level of poverty, and of mortality due to epilepsy-induced accidents.

Prof. David Molyneux, a leading advocate for NTDs and helminthic control programmes, has said "… if you are going to do anything about the MDGs, which have the overall objective of taking people out of poverty, then you had better do something about the diseases which affect the most people rather than those that affect the minority" (8). Thus, the control of high-burden NTDs in low- and middle-income countries will depend on sustainable, although not indefinite, external financial assistance. Global financing mechanisms for NTDs should take into consideration that disease control programmes must be nationally owned, embedded in national health plans, and backed by political commitment, possibly by institutionalizing the recognition and control of these diseases within national education and health programmes.

Another major issue that affects significantly the capacity of several nations to reach the MDGs is the lack of trained human resources, or, when individuals have been trained, an inadequate environment for them to tackle health problems within a research culture. Although some countries are in the process of overcoming these difficulties, and several high-level meetings on health research have called for action in this respect (Mexico City, Abuja, Accra, Algiers and more recently Bamako), a clear commitment has not yet been made by all participating nations. In Bamako, during the Call to Action 2009 meeting, all stakeholders were urged to "promote and share the discovery and development of, and access to, products and technologies addressing neglected and emerging diseases which disproportionately affect low- and middle-income countries". In countries where NTDs are endemic however, different levels of commitment to their resolution occur.

1.2 Human helminthiases, populations at risk and resulting diseases

The helminth infections covered in this report are: onchocerciasis, lymphatic filariasis, soil-transmitted helminthiases, schistosomiasis, food-borne trematodiases and taeniasis/cysticercosis.

Helminth parasites are parasitic worms from the phyla Nematoda (roundworms) and Platyhelminthes (flatworms). Together, they comprise the most common infectious agents of humans in developing countries. The most common helminthiases of humans are those caused by infection with the STHs causing ascariasis, trichuriasis, and hookworm infection (necatoriasis, ancylostomiasis), followed by schistosomiasis and LF. Table 1 summarizes for each condition the estimated number of people infected (although estimates are given separately, there is a significant amount of co-infection), the burden of disease (in terms of disability-adjusted life-years or DALYs), and the estimated number of annual deaths attributable to each disease. The collective burden of the common helminth diseases rivals that of the main high-mortality conditions such as HIV/AIDS or malaria; 85% of the NTD burden for the poorest 500 million people living in sub-Saharan Africa results from helminth infections. Of the 580 million people in Latin America and the Caribbean, 241 million live in areas where at least one of the NTDs is endemic (*9, 10*). Since the remit of this report is centered on the issue of identifying research priorities for the improvement of helminth control programmes, the infections are ordered not in terms of their abundance but in terms of their history of intervention, with the OCP in West Africa (1975–2002) being the first large-scale programme to have been initiated (originally based on vector control).

Onchocerciasis affects 37 million people in 34 countries and is the second cause of infectious blindness after trachoma, with 99% of the cases in SSA. In Latin America and the Caribbean, onchocerciasis has been endemic in Mexico, Guatemala, Colombia, Ecuador, Venezuela and Brazil, with 13 focal areas and 510 000 individuals at risk of infection (*14*); for eight focal areas there is evidence of interruption of transmission (*9, 10*), and Colombia has declared elimination. In onchocerciasis, morbidity is manifested as ocular involvement including blindness, skin disease, palpable nodules, neuro-hormonal involvement including associations with epilepsy and hypo-sexual dwarfism (Nakalanga syndrome), and lymphatic involvement including lymphadenopathy, hanging groin, and lymphoedema. Although onchocercal ocular disease and blindness are more prominent in savannah regions, onchodermatitis or onchocercal skin disease (OSD) has a higher prevalence in forest areas, possibly because of differences in strains of the causal agent, *Onchocerca volvulus*. The importance of OSD as a contributor to the disease burden of onchocerciasis has been recognized relatively recently (*15*).

Table 1
The worldwide abundance, burden of disease, distribution, and control / elimination programmes of human helminthiases (modified from (2, 3, 11))

Infection	Causal agent	Region with highest no. infected	Number infected (millions)	DALYs (millions)	Number of deaths/year (thousands)	Programmes involved
Onchocerciasis	Onchocerca volvulus	SSA	37	1.5[a]	0.05 (in the OCP area)[b] <500	OCP, APOC, OEPA
Lymphatic filariasis	Wuchereria bancrofti; Brugia malayi	India, SEA, SSA	120	5.8	<500	GPELF
Ascariasis	Ascaris lumbricoides	Asia, Africa, LA	1221–1,472[c]	1.8–10.5[c]	3–60[c]	PPC, DtW, GPELF, SCI, CWW
Trichuriasis	Trichuris trichiura	Asia, Africa, LA	759–1050[c]	1.0–6.4[c]	3–10[c]	PPC, DtW, GPELF, SCI, CWW
Hookworm infection	Necator americanus; Ancylostoma duodenale	Asia, Africa, LA	740–1300[c]	0.1–22.1[c]	3–65[c]	PPC, DtW, GPELF, SCI, CWW
Schistosomiasis	Schistosoma mansoni S. haematobium S. japonicum	SSA, LA SSA PRC, SEA	207	1.7–4.5[c]	15–280[c]	SCI in SSA; national programmes elsewhere

continues

Table 1 continued

Infection	Causal agent	Region with highest no. infected	Number infected (millions)	DALYs (millions)	Number of deaths/year (thousands)	Programmes involved
Food-borne trematodiases	*Clonorchis sinensis*; *Opisthorchis viverrini*; *Paragonimus* spp.; *Fasciolopsis buski*; *Fasciola hepatica*	East Asia	56[d]	0.5–0.9[d]	7[d]	Large-scale control initiatives are lacking
Cestode infections: cysticercosis	*Taenia solium*	SSA, Asia, LA	0.4 (LA only)	ND	ND	Large-scale control initiatives are lacking

SSA: Sub-Saharan Africa; PRC: People's Republic of China; SEA: South-East Asia; LA: Latin America.
OCP: Onchocerciasis Control Programme in West Africa (1975–2002); APOC: African Programme for Onchocerciasis Control (1995–ongoing); OEPA: Onchocerciasis Elimination Program for the Americas (1993–ongoing); GPELF: Global Program to Eliminate Lymphatic Filariasis (2002–ongoing); PPC: Partners for Parasite Control (2001–ongoing); DtW: Deworm the World (2007–ongoing); SCI: Schistosomiasis Control Initiative (2002–ongoing); CWW: Children Without Worms (2009–ongoing); ND: not determined.
[a] From Remme et al. *(12)*.
[b] From Little et al. *(13)*.
[c] From Utzinger and Keiser *(534)*.
[d] From Fürst et al. *(535)*.

Lymphatic filariasis is endemic in 83 countries and territories. It is estimated that 1.3 billion people are at risk of developing the disease and some 120 million people are infected. Over 40 million patients are seriously incapacitated and disfigured by the disease. Of these, 95% are infected with *Wuchereria bancrofti*, and the remainder with *Brugia malayi* or *Brugia timori* (*16*). The disease, usually acquired in early childhood, causes considerable morbidity and social stigma because of the deformities it produces. LF provokes acute dermatolymphangioadenitis (ADLA) and lymphoedema. Major chronic manifestations include hydrocoele and lymphoedema of limbs as well as chyluria, lymphoedema of scrotum, adenopathy, haematuria and tropical pulmonary eosinophilia. The disease causes permanent and long-term disability, damages and deforms the limbs, breasts and genitals, in addition to serious psychosocial consequences. Worldwide, 5 million DALYs are lost annually due to LF. The South-East Asia Region accounts for about 57% of the total global burden. India's losses due to LF have been estimated at US$ 1 billion per year.

The STHs are among the most common and persistent parasitic infections worldwide. According to the latest estimates, 800 million people are infected with roundworm (*Ascaris lumbricoides*), 600 million with whipworm (*Trichuris trichiura*), and 600 million with hookworm (*Necator americanus*, *Ancylostoma duodenale*). Although not mentioned further in this report, it is worth noting that 30–100 million people are thought to be infected with threadworm (*Strongyloides stercoralis*) (*3*). In Latin America and the Caribbean, STHs are present in all countries, with an estimated 26.3 million school-aged children at risk of infection. In many areas of 13 of the 14 countries in this region, infection prevalence is higher than 20% (*9, 10, 17*). Globally, approximately 300 million people suffer from severe morbidity, resulting in 10 000–135 000 deaths annually. However, the greatest impact of STHs is on the impairment of physical and mental development in children, which ultimately retards educational advancement and economic development. The relationship between hookworm infection and anaemia is well recognized, with numerous intervention trials showing that a direct effect of cure of infection is reduction in prevalence and intensity of iron deficiency anaemia. However, for *A. lumbricoides* and *T. trichiura* infection, the relationship between infection and specific morbidity measures is less well established. The uncommon, but potentially severe adverse clinical outcomes of rectal prolapse due to *T. trichiura* infection and bile duct or intestinal obstruction due to *A. lumbricoides* infection are well recognized in the medical literature. However, there is a lack of epidemiological data defining the prevalence of these complications, and relating them to community prevalence and infection intensity (*18–20*). Less easily measured parameters such as hypoproteinaemia have been attributed to heavy infection with these parasites, but likewise there is a dearth of quality epidemiological data. Studies have been undertaken to relate school, cognitive, and athletic performance to infection, largely through chemotherapy interventions. While there appears to be some effect, distinguishing this from other coexisting confounding variables such as micro- and macronutrient deficiency is not straightforward.

Schistosomiasis is endemic in 76 countries and territories in the tropics and subtropics. *Schistosoma mansoni* is endemic in 54 countries and *S. haematobium* in 55 (*21*). Infection by *S. japonicum* remains an important public health burden in the Philippines, the People's Republic of China (PRC) and parts of Indonesia, despite continued efforts by ongoing control programmes (*22*). Worldwide, almost 800 million individuals are at risk; about 200 million people are estimated to be infected, and most of these suffer some level of morbidity (*23–25*). Of the 200 million people infected, 160 million live in SSA, where approximately 110 million are infected with *S. haematobium* (*26*). Schistosomiasis causes 150 000–280 000 deaths annually in SSA alone (*26*), and severe disability in approximately 20 million people. In its chronic stage the disease leads to portal hypertension and organomegaly in 5%–8% of untreated infections, and it is also strongly associated with liver and bladder cancers.

S. haematobium infection is particularly burdensome, causing a large number of cases of hydronephrosis, renal failure, and bladder cancer. Women with urinary schistosomiasis have an increased risk of HIV infection. Over 80% of the schistosomiasis burden is concentrated in SSA. In Latin America and the Caribbean, schistosomiasis (mansoni) is prevalent in Brazil, Suriname and Venezuela, with 25 million people at risk of infection and 1–3 million people infected. The figures presented in Table 1 (corresponding to the Global Burden of Disease estimates for 2000 and updated in 2004) are thought to considerably underestimate the true burden of schistosomiasis (*27, 28*). As for almost all helminth infections, schistosome infection is not equivalent to schistosomiasis disease. Likewise, there is a paucity of validated direct and indirect indicators of schistosome-related morbidity (*29–32*). In urinary schistosomiasis, gross haematuria is an obvious early visual sign of morbidity; however, for *S. mansoni* and *S. japonicum*, assessment of morbidity is more difficult. Furthermore, few, if any, of the clinical manifestations of schistosomiasis are specific, being potentially related to other causes, including other helminth infections and malaria, which often co-exist with schistosomiasis.

The human liver flukes, causing infections known as food-borne trematodiases, and including *Opisthorchis viverrini*, *Op. felineus* and *Clonorchis sinensis*, remain important public health problems, particularly in Asia. Chronic infections with *Op. viverrini* and *C. sinensis* have long been associated with cholangiocarcinoma – the bile duct cancer. *C. sinensis* is widespread in PRC, Korea, and the Socialist Republic of Vietnam, while *Op. viverrini* is endemic in South-East Asia, including Thailand, Lao People's Democratic Republic (Lao PDR), Cambodia and central Vietnam. Recent reports suggest that about 35 million people are infected with *C. sinensis* globally, with up to 15 million human infections in PRC alone, and another 10 million individuals infected with *Op. viverrini* in Thailand and Lao PDR. A recent review estimated that 80 million people in Thailand, Lao PDR, Cambodia, Vietnam and Eastern Europe are at risk for infection with *Op. viverrini* and *Op. felineus*. Over 45 million people are infected by the two liver flukes, *Op. viverrini* and *C. sinensis*; more than 600 million people, mainly in Asia and including PRC, Korea, Taiwan, and Vietnam, are at risk of infection (*33*). The infections are associated with hepatobiliary diseases including hepatomegaly, cholangitis, fibrosis of the periportal system, cholecystitis, gallstones, and are major aetiological agents of cholangiocarcinoma. In the liver fluke endemic area of Khon Kaen, North-East Thailand, the highest incidence of this liver cancer in the world has been reported. In addition, liver and bile duct cancers, end-stage consequences of liver fluke disease, ranked number five in Thai males and number six in females among all diseases with the highest number of DALYs in 2005.

Taenia solium is endemic in Latin America, vast parts of Asia including PRC and the Indian subcontinent, Eastern Europe and most of Africa. Imported cases occur in most developed countries due to immigration from and tourism to endemic regions. The *T. solium* taeniasis/cysticercosis complex involves two different life-stage and clinical entities affecting the human host. Taeniasis, the intestinal infection by the adult tapeworm (when humans act as definitive host), causes low morbidity by itself but represents the sole source of cysticercosis infection to humans and pigs. Cysticercosis, the infection with the larval stage of the parasite or cysticercus (when humans act as intermediate host), is a major cause of seizure disorders worldwide (human neurocysticercosis or NCC) and also causes economic losses due to infected pork (porcine cysticercosis). The most consistent indicator is the frequency of neurocysticercosis in individuals with seizure disorders. In several endemic areas of Latin America the attributed fraction for NCC is around 30% of all seizure disorders. Subarachnoid NCC is also associated with intracranial hypertension and mortality.

Control of *S. japonicum* and cestode infections in humans is also complicated by the fact that they constitute zoonotic infections. As indicated in the DRG6 report, other animals e.g. cattle, buffalo, rodents, dogs, sheep and pigs can act as reservoirs for human transmission of *S. japonicum*. The control effort of *S. japonicum* in the People's Republic of China is fully addressed in the DGR6 report. Additionally, a pilot study for integrated control of schistosomiasis has been undertaken in PRC using a multi-pronged approach ranging from the removal of bovines from snail-infested grassland to the supply of tap water as well as intensive health education (DRG6 report). In the case of cestodes, and also schistosomiasis despite the proven use of praziquantel (PZQ), there is need for improved drugs and/or studies with drug combination regimens and dosages to evaluate their efficacy and reduce the risk of transmission (see DRG6 report for fuller details).

Epidemiologically, human helminthiases are characterized by long-lasting infections with more than one helminth species. This phenomenon, known as polyparasitism, is the result of commonalities in ecological and environmental requirements, infection routes, host exposures and susceptibility, as well as behavioural, sociological, and economic factors that enable co-occurrence of a multiplicity of parasite-host systems in time and space. In Figure 1, the geographical distribution of co-occurrence of lymphatic filariasis, onchocerciasis, schistosomiasis and STHs at country level is presented. While the prevalence of human neurocysticercosis (NCC) worldwide remains unknown, initiatives are currently under way to determine the burden of NCC in endemic countries of Africa, Asia and Latin America (*34–36*) as well as in industrialized countries such as the USA where it is becoming a growing problem because of immigration of tapeworm carriers from endemic areas. As the estimate for proportion of NCC among people with epilepsy is very robust (*36*), it could be used, in conjunction with estimates of the prevalence and incidence of epilepsy, to estimate this component of the burden of NCC in endemic areas.

As studies have demonstrated that individuals with multiple helminthiases may also have the most intense infections (*37–41*), polyparasitism may have a greater impact on morbidity than the sum of single-species infections. In addition, multiple species infections may increase susceptibility to other infections such as malaria or HIV (*42, 43*), particularly given the immunosuppresive nature of helminth infections. Consequently, efforts have been made to better understand the consequences of the co-existence of parasites within the same host on the immunological responses to each species and, more importantly, whether such interactions affect resistance, susceptibility or clinical outcome (*44*). Co-infections are also shifting some of the prevention and control measures of helminth infections from single-drug treatments to integrated approaches that can simultaneously target as many as four of the helminth neglected tropical diseases, including onchocerciasis, LF, STHs, and schistosomiasis – a mission undertaken by the GNNTDC and the WHO (*2, 4*).

1.3 Group membership

The Disease Reference Group on Helminth Infections (DRG4) consists of 13 experts in the area of helminth infections and its cross-cutting themes (Annex 2). Members were identified from research institutions, international organizations, bilateral institutions, health and medical organizations, and governmental and inter-governmental organizations worldwide. Particular attention was paid to the geographical distribution, to ensure disease-endemic country representation and regional input as well as technical input, and gender balance of the membership. Members were formally appointed by the Director, TDR, for an initial period of two years. All members were obliged to declare any conflict of interest and confidentiality.

Introduction

Figure 1
Geographic distribution of co-infections with helminths – lymphatic filariasis (LF), onchocerciasis (Oncho), schistosomiasis (SCH), soil-transmitted helminthiases (STH) – in 2009 (45)

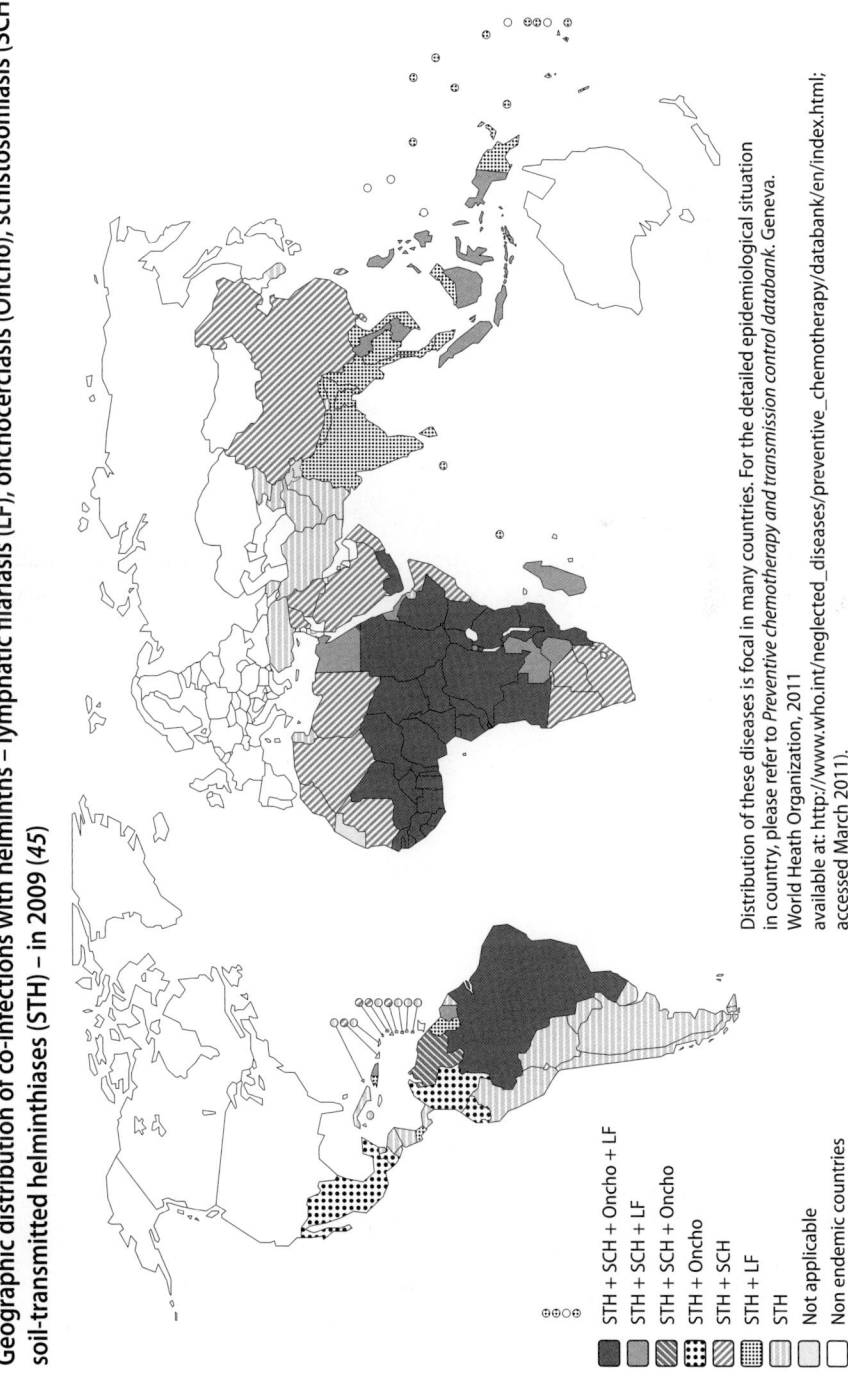

Distribution of these diseases is focal in many countries. For the detailed epidemiological situation in country, please refer to *Preventive chemotherapy and transmission control databank*. Geneva. World Heath Organization, 2011 available at: http://www.who.int/neglected_diseases/preventive_chemotherapy/databank/en/index.html; accessed March 2011).

STH + SCH + Oncho + LF
STH + SCH + LF
STH + SCH + Oncho
STH + Oncho
STH + SCH
STH + LF
STH
Not applicable
Non endemic countries

The chair and co-chair of the group were selected on the basis of their internationally-recognized research and control experience in disease-endemic countries.

1.4 Host country

To ensure that the countries most affected by diseases of poverty contribute to, and share ownership of, the research agenda emerging from this initiative, the reference groups are hosted by disease-endemic countries, in partnership with WHO country and regional offices (Annex 1).

The Disease Reference Group on Helminth Infections (DRG4) was hosted in APOC headquarters, Ouagadougou, Burkina Faso.

1.5 TDR Think Tank members

The TDR Think Tank was designed to draw on the best expertise internationally (Annex 3), and to maximize partnerships with countries most affected by diseases of poverty. The ten reference groups making up the Think Tank include researchers and public health experts from the most affected countries, and these countries also host the groups. WHO country and regional offices support both the reference groups and broad-based stakeholder consultations (Annex 4).

2. Methodology and prioritization

This part of the report sets out the methods used to identify the research priorities in relation to helminth infections. These included the identification of which helminthiases to consider, conceptualization and preparation of white papers on specific topics, prioritization of research areas and recommendations, and validation of the prepared annual report. A multistage process as set out below was used to arrive at the final product.

2.1 Identification of the helminth infections to be considered

A group of renowned scientists with experience in infectious diseases of poverty were brought together for a consultation by TDR, the Special Programme for Research and Training in Tropical Diseases, to recommend experts to consider research needs in this area. The group arrived at the following: 1) nomination of 13 experts in helminth infections – the Disease Reference Group on Helminth Infections (DRG4) (Annex 2); 2) helminth infections to be considered by DRG4; and 3) suggestions of areas where research is needed.

The helminth infections recommended to be covered were: onchocerciasis, lymphatic filariasis, soil-transmitted helminthiases, schistosomiasis, food-borne trematodiases and taeniasis/cysticercosis.

The 13 topics below were recommended for discussion:

1. Knowledge on the current situation of helminthic diseases worldwide
2. Requirements to achieve control and elimination
3. Epidemiology including diagnostic tools
4. Issues of sustainability, advocacy, and human resources
5. Data availability, surveillance and drug resistance
6. Discovery and research on new drugs (natural products, new formulations, production)
7. Basic research (immune mechanisms, genome/genomics)
8. Vaccine development as part of integrated prevention and/or immunotherapy
9. Data management and sharing
10. Drug availability
11. Availability of diagnostic kits
12. Access to treatment and health care
13. Pre-clinical and clinical trials.

A concept note that included the mandate, activities and rationale for DRG4, a plan of work and timelines for producing a first annual report on research priorities in helminth infections was developed and circulated for review, validation and full agreement by members of DRG4. Members were asked to obtain, evaluate and synthesize scientific information on current activities in global research on helminth infections, highlight progress, identify knowledge gaps, needs and the challenges faced, and suggest priorities for future global research based on four questions:

- What is known
- What research has not been used or applied
- What is not known
- What research is needed.

2.2 Identification of the research gaps to be considered

Each DRG4 member was asked to prepare, based on his/her specific area of expertise, one or more white papers based on the above 13 topics (section 2.1), and to identify and list the research gaps. The white papers were circulated between members for comment, and later presented orally and discussed at the first meeting of the DRG4, hosted in Ouagadougou, Burkina Faso, by the African Programme for Onchocerciasis Control (APOC) and the WHO Regional Office for Africa.

The topics of the white papers were:

1. Anti-helminth vaccines as part of the solution to control helminthic infections of poverty
2. Operations research, challenges and needs to help fill programmatic gaps: *O. volvulus* and lymphatic filariae
3. Community-directed intervention: successes, issues, challenges and needs
4. Surveillance for sub-optimal response by *Onchocerca volvulus* to ivermectin
5. New drugs and new treatments for onchocerciasis and lymphatic filariasis
6. Operational studies/challenges to control/prevent liver fluke infections/diseases with particular emphasis on those unique to South-East Asia
7. Control of schistosomiasis: strategies and challenges
8. Epidemiological, entomological, and parasitological patterns of helminth infections

9. The role mathematical models can play in parasite control, elimination, monitoring and evaluation, and surveillance
10. Taeniasis/cysticercosis: epidemiology and impact, diagnosis, treatment, control tools and status
11. Are the strategies for the implementation of polyparasitism control programmes adequate and widely available for use by disease-endemic countries?
12. Anthelmintic discovery
13. Current diagnostic techniques for monitoring efficacy of mass drug administration (MDA) programmes for soil-transmitted helminths (STH) and other helminth infections: limitations, and needs for improvement, of existing tools and/or the development of new tools
14. Geospatial tools for disease risk mapping, surveillance and predictions for resource allocation in order to achieve the goals of integrated and sustainable control of helminthiases
15. MDA control measures and potential emergence of drug resistance, including gaps in surveillance and genetic assays (*O. volvulus*, *W. bancrofti* and STHs)
16. New integrated strategies to control transmission of schistosomiasis, including lessons from the People's Republic of China and South-East Asia
17. Influence of climate and environmental change on disease burden and control measures
18. Preventative chemotherapy and transmission control: issues related to research in the field of helminthiases
19. Addressing resistance development in tropical disease pathogens
20. Life-cycle management and pharmacoepidemiology.

2.3 The first DRG4 meeting

The first DRG4 meeting was immediately preceded by the first national and local stakeholder's consultation, with the aim to obtain input and suggestions on the priority research areas for helminth infections. These suggestions were discussed, along with those from the TDR expert consultation members (see 2.1), at the first meeting of the DRG4 in January 2010.

At the meeting, five core themes were identified as umbrella priorities to support the control and elimination of helminthiases: intervention, epidemiology and surveillance, environmental and social ecology, data and modelling, and basic (fundamental) biology (Figure 2). Priorities within these umbrella themes were also identified.

Figure 2
The five major core themes identified as umbrella priorities to support the control and elimination of the helminthiases under the remit of DRG4

GLOBAL, REGIONAL, NATIONAL, LOCAL	Filariases (onchocerciasis, lymphatic filariasis); soil-transmitted helminthiases; schistosomiasis and other trematodiases; cestode infections	(1) INTERVENTIONS	Optimize existing/develop novel methods (drugs, vaccines, anti-vector measures) for control of helminth infection and transmission to help reduce the duration of control/elimination programmes so as to maximize commitment and sustainability and minimize polyparasitism and development of resistance
		(2) EPIDEMIOLOGY AND SURVEILLANCE	Improve existing/develop novel diagnostic assays for monitoring and evaluation of the impact of control programmes on helminth infection and associated morbidity, and for supporting decisions towards control/ elimination end-points. Optimize existing/ develop novel instruments for effective surveillance, including prompt detection of resistance, pharmacovigilance, and post-intervention surveillance systems.
		(3) ENVIRONMENT AND SOCIAL ECOLOGY	Strengthen understanding of the sociological, behavioural, political and economic drivers of helminth infection and control to: improve community knowledge/education; achieve empowerment/equity/gender, participation and ownership; and increase intervention coverage, compliance and sustainability.
		(4) DATA AND MODELLING	Continuously update and share data platforms to optimize data management, analysis, and (mathematical/statistical/geographical/climate change) modelling, integrating scientists, stakeholders and end-users.
		(5) BIOLOGY	Conduct studies on the pathogenesis, genetics, population structure, vector–parasite–host(s) interactions and immunology to further support the basis for translating basic research into operations/implementation of existing or improved control measures.

ADVOCACY, INTEGRATION AND INNOVATION

Five sub-groups were formed, one for each of the five core themes, to provide: 1) an overview of trends and driving forces of persistent, emerging and re-emerging helminth infections and the consequential research and control challenges; 2) an overview of significant recent scientific advances; 3) a deeper analysis of control challenges/ research issues by particular disease/risk factors; and 4) a gap analysis and identification of research priorities.

The sub-groups reviewed their reports to arrive at consensus on the priority research issues and recommendations pertaining to the core theme. The five sub-group reports were later compiled into a single DRG4 draft report by the chairpersons and various DRG4 members comprising the core writing team in New York, April 2010.

2.4 Prioritization of themes

Deeper analysis of the 35 identified research gaps, and electronic exchange of reports, led to the identification of 40 main topics (research areas) and 90 sub-topics for research and recommendations, based on the following values and criteria for ranking.

2.4.1 Underlying values

- Curative or preventative relevance at patient/community level
- Public health relevance/impact on population health
- Pro-poor/poverty alleviating
- Related to millennium development goals (MDGs) and/or other global targets
- Health security relevance
- Intersectoral
- Equity/gender equity/social justice
- Positive risk–benefit ratio
- Feasibility
- Universality
- Global public good
- Innovation.

2.4.2 Criteria for ranking

- Potential public health impact (by disease burden reduction)
- Size of population benefiting from research
- Feasibility (cost benefit)

- Economic implications (cost effectiveness)
- Equity implications
- Equality implications.

The first full draft report of DRG4, with 90 research areas within five core themes (Figure 2), was reviewed in detail by each member of the group, and their comments incorporated into a subsequent, second draft of the report. The second draft, with unranked priority research issues and recommendations was then reviewed by the chairs and co-chairs of the other DRGs and thematic reference groups (TRGs), and their comments taken into consideration in preparing a subsequent, third draft report.

This third draft report was presented at a second stakeholder's consultation in Rio de Janeiro, Brazil, in October 2010 for comments and suggestions as well as for arriving at a consensus on the final research priorities.

2.5 The second DRG4 meeting

At the second meeting of the DRG4, held in Rio de Janeiro, Brazil, immediately following the stakeholder's consultation meeting, the final selection and ranking of the priority research areas as well as the practical timelines for each research activity were determined as outlined below. Following extensive discussion, the group came to an agreement on 26 research priorities (section 8) for the five umbrella themes that would enable progress in the field of helminthiasis control and identification of novel tools to eliminate the public health problem posed by these infections or their reservoirs.

2.6 Ranking of priority research areas by experts in DRG4

Each DRG4 member independently ranked the 26 priority research areas within the five core themes and also between the six helminthiases, guided by the underlying values and criteria for ranking listed above, scoring them from 1 to 5, with 5 corresponding to the highest priority. They also set hypothetical time frames for the achievement of each of the priority areas identified, in time horizons of 5-, 10-, 15-, 20- and 25-year periods. Based on the means of the scores from each DRG4 member, the two research areas with the highest mean scores within each of the five core themes were then selected to provide the ten top priority research areas (Box 1, page xvii). A league table was prepared for the ten priority research areas using the individual scores as criteria, as indicated in Annex 5.

For the priority research areas, the time frames provided by DRG4 members were collated into periods of 1–5 years (short term), 5–15 years (medium term) and 15–25 years (long term). These timelines were used to project the impact that completion of the research landmarks would have on the helminthiases in the short, medium and long terms, as well as on the achievement of the MDGs, taking into consideration their impacts also on technological innovation, health systems and the environment, as presented in Annex 6.

2.7 Stakeholders consultation meetings and other external contributions

Periodic regional and national stakeholder consultations are an essential part of the analysis process, enabling validation, endorsement and uptake of final research priorities, and ensuring that the work is authoritative, scientifically credible, and relevant for policy. Below are specific details about the stakeholders and the stakeholder consultation meetings.

Two stakeholder consultations were held, the first immediately prior to the first meeting of DRG4 and the second after the draft report had been completed.

2.7.1 First stakeholders' consultation

The first stakeholder consultation was held at the African Programme for Onchocerciasis Control (APOC) headquarters, Ouagadougou, Burkina Faso, in January 2010. The Ministry of Health/Burkina Faso, Helen Keller International, RISEAL/Burkina Faso, United Nations Children's Fund (UNICEF) office, WHO/Multi Disease Surveillance Center (MDSC), the WHO Country Office and WHO/APOC were represented. Presentations from the stakeholders regarding their perspective of the research gaps and needs were given and included with those identified by the DRG4 committee members. The lists of the gaps identified were formatted into a slide presentation, reviewed and discussed until 35 core areas were obtained.

2.7.2 Second stakeholders' consultation

The second stakeholder consultation took place in Rio de Janeiro, Brazil, on 8 October 2010. Participants included representatives of the Ministry of Health of Brazil, WHO/PAHO, researchers from Oswaldo Cruz Institute (Rio de Janeiro), and other international and local experts attending the International Schistosomiasis Symposium in Rio de Janeiro, 5–8 October 2010. Five members of the DRG4 presented a summary of the Group's mission and the research priorities identified in each of the five core themes. The participants provided their comments and validation of the draft report and recommendations of DRG4; their input and suggestions were subsequently discussed at the second DRG4 meeting held in Rio de Janeiro, 9–10 October 2010.

Additionally, the DRG4 obtained feedback from regional committees in Brazil, South-East Asia and Latin America, who reviewed the research priorities in their own regions. Notably, their priorities (46–49) were largely in agreement with those arrived at by DRG4.

2.8 Publication of the DRG4 report

The process of finalization of the report and its transformation into a publication of the WHO Technical Report Series was carried out through electronic communication between the Chair, co-Chair, DRG members and the Secretariat. The Secretariat undertook the organization of external and internal reviews of the Report, and comments on structure and content were addressed in the final version of the Report.

This Report was assessed by the WHO Guidelines Review Committee, which recommended that it be published as an Expert Report.

3. Overview of trends and driving forces of persistent, emerging and re-emerging helminth infections and the consequent research and control challenges

3.1 Parasite population biology and human host sociological factors

Epidemiologically, human helminthiases are characterized by long-lasting infection with one or, more often, more than one of the helminth species referred to above. This phenomenon, known as polyparasitism, is the result of commonalities in ecological and environmental requirements, infection routes, host exposures and susceptibility, as well as behavioural, sociological, and economic factors that enable co-occurrence of a multiplicity of parasite-host systems in time and space. Infection prevalence at any time-point may be high and this, in addition to reflecting a high intensity of transmission, also reflects the long duration of some infections – parasites may have a long life-span, while hosts do not recover, do not mount effective infection-clearing immune responses, and are exposed to repeated infection throughout their lives.

Further, aggregation of infection, whereby a minority of individuals harbours very heavy infection but the majority of the population harbours light or moderate infection, is a major factor to consider in epidemiological studies, chemotherapy efficacy trials, and in efforts to reduce prevalence, if for example "wormy" individuals are somehow missed in drug treatment programmes.

Among the biological determinants of persisting infection is the fact that parasite populations are strongly regulated within their hosts (both definitive and intermediate, including vector and snail hosts), which makes them highly stable and resilient to control interventions. Therefore, premature cessation of interventions may lead to re-emergence and eventual restoration of the parasite population to baseline levels. Among the sociological factors contributing to this stability are those that link infection, particularly heavy infection, with chronic and long-lasting morbidity, disability, insidious and irreversible effects on health, poor school performance, impaired ability to work, low economic productivity, and premature death. All this perpetuates the vicious circle that links helminthiases to poverty, lack of sanitation, poor hygiene, and marginalization.

All of the above points towards shifting the paradigm from single to multi-disease and integrated approaches to the prevention and control of helminth infection. There is also a need to develop indicators capable of capturing meaningful impacts of multiple interventions, such as reduced anaemia, improved school attendance, and increased labour productivity, as well as a need to evaluate the cost–effectiveness of such interventions.

3.2 Chemotherapeutic factors

The majority of the control programmes listed in Table 1, page 7 rely heavily on anthelmintic treatment, and overall have achieved good results with regard to effecting reductions on the prevalence and intensity of infection and morbidity in some endemic areas (*50–53*). Interruption of transmission for some infections, leading towards local elimination, has been reported in some foci (*54–57*). Those programmes which have followed cohorts of individuals longitudinally from the beginning of the interventions, have also allowed changes in the incidence of infection and/or morbidity to be assessed (*58, 59*).

One reason for this heavy reliance on chemotherapy is because the drugs are donated by pharmaceutical companies for some programmes, or their cost has become affordable (*2*). Chemotherapy may represent a rapid-impact package because the impact of anthelmintic treatment on parasite populations is proportionally largest at the beginning of the intervention, but long-term sustainability of the benefits accrued will critically depend on altering the environmental components that facilitate transmission. Large-scale elimination of the infection reservoir will depend on improving sanitation and drainage, providing access to clean water, adequately disposing of excreta and solid waste, promoting access to health services for diagnosis and treatment, and facilitating adequate housing and health education (*60, 61*). Hopefully, anthelmintic treatment can be seen as a necessary, but not sufficient, condition towards breaking the vicious circle between helminth infection, ill-health and chronic poverty.

Anthelmintic treatment can be distributed using a variety of treatment strategies, depending on the level of infection endemicity, the overall aim of the control programme (elimination of the public health burden or of the infection reservoir), the population groups which exhibit the highest infection levels, and the relationship between infection and disease sequelae (for morbidity control). Treatment can be aimed at particular occupational or age groups (such as school-age children) most at risk of acquiring heavy infection and severe morbidity. This is the basis for school-based health programmes aimed at deworming children of STHs and schistosomiasis. In this target population, treatment is administered to all eligible individuals regardless of whether or not they are patently infected. In areas of substantial endemicity, community (mass) treatment is recommended. Other strategies include mass screen and treat (MSAT) (targeting selective treatment to those with patent and detectable infection), or treating individual cases in clinical as opposed to community settings. The adoption of such treatment modalities may also depend on the stage of the control programme, with mass drug administration (MDA) being implemented at its commencement, and selective treatment in the mopping-up phases. Those programmes which aim at eliminating the infection reservoir will tend to treat the largest number of people with the highest possible coverage for as long as autochthonous transmission persists, and this may impose strong selection pressures upon parasite genomes, affecting genetic diversity and favouring drug resistant strains. This could lead to resurgence of infection in areas previously under control.

Optimum treatment coverage MDA is required for the success of control and elimination programmes for helminthic infections. Models predict, and experience confirms, that population coverage is a key determinant of the success of such programmes and there is still a need to evaluate the compliance of the population in participating in such programmes over the years. The use of the term 'therapeutic coverage' implies that the persons who receive the drugs are actually taking them (i.e. they are compliant), but in several countries, most notably India, a gap between coverage and compliance has been observed in the case of lymphatic filariasis (LF) (62, 63). The contribution of non-compliant persons to transmission is unknown, but systematic non-compliance may represent a potential threat for helminth control or elimination. Furthermore, the sustainability of the required long-term treatment programmes also raises issues of compliance related to possible population fatigue, waning interest of community drug distributors, and funding, as the original funds from external donors used to initiate the treatment-based control programmes may be time-limited.

Deeper analyses of host sociological factors, and factors affecting access to health services, are covered by the reports of the Thematic Reference Groups on Social Sciences and Gender (TRG1) and Health Systems and Implementation Research (TRG3). This Disease Reference Group 4 (DRG4) report cross-references TRG1 with respect to host social factors in the chemotherapy of helminthiases. Important factors in chemotherapy are gender sensitiveness and targeting of specific age groups, e.g. school age and occupational groups. The TRG1 report also looks at the issues of free vs. paid-for interventions and other social issues in detail. The cross reference of DRG4 to TRG3 is best indicated in section 5.4 of this report.

3.3 Factors associated with current ability to diagnose helminth infections in individuals, communities and larger spatial scales

The technical limitations of available diagnostic methods for helminthiases impose significant constraints on current initiatives to control these infections. Appropriate diagnostic methodologies are required for: disease mapping to guide initiation of interventions; case-based diagnosis; monitoring and evaluation (M&E) of intervention programmes, particularly with the possible threat of failure of the interventions due to technical reasons (including drug resistance and other selective pressures imposed upon parasite and vector populations e.g.

immune selection leading to vaccine escape mutants, and insecticide resistance in vectors); determining when an intervention can be safely ended in the setting of elimination to confirm interruption of transmission; epidemiological surveillance in post-control areas, and areas where elimination may have been certified.

For each of these activities the technical requirements for diagnostic tests are likely to be different and possibly represent different technical challenges. Furthermore, our ability to diagnose infection status differs for each of the helminth species considered here due to the different biology of the parasites (life-cycle, accessibility to parasitological diagnosis, body fluid appropriate for sampling, role of and need to sample vector or intermediate hosts) and of the parasite-host systems (including age profiles of infection prevalence and intensity). In addition, intensity of infection is a critical determinant of morbidity and disease burden, and as described above, is also critical for the stability of the host-parasite relationship, contribution to density-dependent, regulatory mechanisms of parasite population abundance, and contribution to transmission. Yet, with few exceptions this critical parameter is difficult to quantify with present tools.

Not only is the diagnosis of individual infections important, but also it is essential to understand the spatial distribution of infections within countries and communities, as well as within the individual. The effectiveness of large-scale integrated programmes for the control of neglected tropical diseases (NTDs) in general, and helminth diseases in particular, will depend on the geographical overlap between the different NTDs. In spite of being co-endemic in particular countries (64), different NTDs can, in certain settings, exhibit limited geographical overlap at sub-national scales, necessitating a more geographically-targeted approach for integrated NTD control (60, 65). A major obstacle to the implementation of cost-effective control is the lack of accurate descriptions of the geographical distribution of infection. In recent years, considerable progress has been made in the use of geographical information systems (GIS) and remote sensing (RS) to better understand helminth ecology and epidemiology, and to develop low-cost and minimally invasive ways to identify target populations for treatment such as the development of methods for rapid epidemiological assessment (REA) of infection and morbidity (66, 67). A major concern is that there is not enough accurate information on the distribution of infection prevalence and intensity to build such maps. In the People's Republic of China (PRC) and Africa predictive maps have been prepared to identify risk areas and help governments and health services plan control strategies. However, the potential of NTD mapping has been less exploited in Latin America (see (68) for rapid epidemiological assessment (REA) methods and (69) for GIS and onchocerciasis in the Amazonian focus). Thus, research is required to determine the optimal strategy for rapidly and simultaneously assessing a number of NTDs so that more effective implementation of integrated approaches for disease control can take place. Reliable and updated maps of helminth infection distributions are essential to target control strategies to those populations in greatest need, and their current lack constitutes a driving force of persisting control challenges. A principal advantage of a GIS platform is that it facilitates the regular updating of information and provides a ready basis for analysis and statistical modelling of spatial distributions (70).

3.4 Factors associated with the environmental and social ecology of human helminthiases

The distribution and burden of helminth infections are not merely a reflection of geographical and ecological circumstances, but also a reflection of the level of political commitment and investment in resources (human, financial) by national governments for the prevention and control of helminthiases in vulnerable populations and the environment they inhabit. Progress in preventing, controlling or eliminating these diseases is slow in some countries. Few health-care systems can guarantee full access to and delivery of the essential medicines for all patients and populations at risk. Most countries have not yet fully taken advantage of the new tools and protocols available for prevention, control and elimination. In order to develop an operative strategy for the prevention and control of NTDs, there is a need to organize public health resources.

For the infections that can be controlled by mass chemotherapy (geohelminthiasis, schistosomiasis), but which may not be readily eliminated, early and intensified case detection and management can be pursued. However, although in some settings mass screen and treat (MSAT) strategies have been implemented, more often than not, after some initial assessment of prevalence and intensity, MDA is implemented, which does not target individual cases of infection. Normally for MDA, clinical services are not required to implement treatment, which can be delivered by community distributors. The widespread epidemiological pattern of helminth infections in endemic countries makes elimination unlikely at present except for limited settings (e.g. the potential to eliminate schistosomiasis in some Caribbean countries).

Surveillance for NTDs should be the responsibility of national and local health authorities. However given the reality that most health-care systems do not yet prioritize surveillance of NTDs, outreach is needed, to involve cooperating health services, health professionals, environmental health officers, and communities who can organize themselves for surveillance.

At a regional, supranational level, a ranking order of the relative importance of NTDs would be difficult to propose. Rankings could be made based on criteria such as presence of global or regional mandates for elimination, magnitude of geographical extension, trends in distribution, and estimated burden of disease. However, it is particularly challenging to establish disease burden due to lack of reliable data for many NTDs as to their incidence, prevalence, intensity, association with morbidity and sequelae, distribution in afflicted populations, and reliable demographic denominators of populations at risk. In any particular country or sub-region it will be necessary to prioritize which NTDs are the most important, based on updated knowledge on local prevalence, disease burden, at risk populations, geographical distribution, and the commitment of governments to equity in health care (coverage and health services goals). In the strategic lines of action to be developed under this framework, a multi-disease, inter-programmatic, and intersectoral approach should be taken wherever scientifically, logistically and economically possible. It should actively seek community involvement with the aim of increasing local empowerment. In this way, the focus of implementation should be through work in partnership with multiple sectors and multiple health programmes. Failure to do so is also a driving force of persisting infection and emerging and re-emerging public health challenges.

3.5 Factors associated with research gaps in basic helminth biology

The main factor associated with the gaps in research on basic helminth biology is the understandable priority given to "applied" or "operational" research at the expense of basic research; "understandable" because of the imperative to better control helminth infections, or to at least relieve the morbidity associated with these infections. The current efforts, based primarily on MDA, have been effective in some cases (e.g. onchocerciasis), and this success has further eroded support for such fundamental research. However, MDA is potentially vulnerable to the development of drug resistance in those cases where chemotherapy has had a major impact on parasite prevalence and transmission (and hence exerts a strong selective pressure), and has suffered from the lack of suitable safe, effective and affordable drugs in other areas. For example, although the macrocyclic lactone ivermectin (IVM) has proved effective in interrupting onchocerciasis transmission in limited settings, no safe and effective macrofilaricide (against adult worms or macrofilariae) for MDA exists; schistosome control critically depends on the sustained clinical efficacy of PZQ; the chemotherapy of many helminth infections is unsatisfactory due to the lack of safe and effective drugs amenable to single dose therapy. Furthermore, there is the potential, at least, for unintended consequences of MDA stemming from the poorly understood dynamics of host-parasite interactions and the effect that altered parasite infection intensity and prevalence may have on those interactions.

What areas of basic research are likely to yield improved control tools? Comparison of helminths with malaria may be instructive in this context:

genomics has transformed malaria research over the past decade, reinvigorating drug and vaccine development, and enabling the development of more sophisticated mathematical models that inform control and elimination efforts. A similar investment in helminth genomics, most particularly in the development of functional tools with which genome sequences can be probed and mined, could catalyse a similar transformation of helminth research.

A major limitation on this front is the limited availability of annotated genome sequences. With the advent of novel rapid and inexpensive genome sequencing technologies, the entire genomes of some selected helminths of medical importance have been successfully sequenced. However, there is a lack of bioinformatic tools, power and reference genomes to accurately annotate them. The genomes of B. malayi, S. mansoni, and S. japonicum have been partially annotated and a low-cost alternative for genome sequencing, expressed sequence tag (EST), has been produced for many helminths, which provide a glimpse of the transcriptome of these species (71–76). However, the complexity of helminth life-cycles, including the various developmental transitions they undergo, makes it a daunting task to understand these transcriptome profiles and, more importantly, the biological role of the genes identified in these studies (77). Functional genomic tools such as RNA interference (RNAi) technology has proved to be useful in deciphering the role of schistosome encoded proteins (78–81). In contrast, RNAi technology has been a largely unsuccessful tool for functional analysis in parasitic nematodes (82, 83). The exact reasons for this are still unclear, but it has been suggested that some essential components of the RNAi pathway are missing in some species (74, 78).

Numerous studies have indicated that helminth-secreted proteins, glycoproteins and lipid-based molecules can interfere with various host immune responses, ultimately leading to the generation of an anti-inflammatory environment, favourable for the parasite's survival (84–86). Some of the processes affected include the development of allergic responses (87, 88) and interference with host cytokine regulation and signal transduction networks (89, 90). These findings highlight the complexity of the biology of helminths with respect to the human/non-human (definitive) hosts and are further complicated by the effects of polyparasitism due to other helminth or protozoan parasites, bacterial or viral infections.

In addition, the importance of endosymbionts of filarial nematodes, especially Wolbachia spp. in B. malayi, W. bancrofti, and O. volvulus, has yet to be fully understood with respect to the ultimate effects on host-parasite interactions (91). Wolbachia spp. undoubtedly confer a survival advantage to B. malayi and other filarial nematodes which enhances their parasitic potential (92, 93). Further exploration of this interaction may lead to development of novel methods of eliminating filarial infections in host populations (94).

Despite the significant advances made in genomic, proteomic and transcriptomic profiles of helminths, these "-omics" are still in their early developmental stages. The influx of bioinformatics knowledge needs to be reconciled with novel research methodologies for functional analysis of genes and the proteins they encode. Since most countries afflicted by helminths are still classified as developing, there is a divide between the available resources for the application of basic research and what is available to scientists in the endemic countries. Thus, the urgency required to explore the incoming wealth of bioinformatics knowledge is skewed towards the few research institutes in Western and developed countries that have funding, which normally has imposed priorities tailored towards the funding agency's interests and not necessarily the actual needs of affected populations and countries (*2*).

4. Overview of significant recent advances for the control and elimination of helminth infections and deeper analysis of control challenges and research issues for helminth diseases

In the last decade, strong evidence-based epidemiological studies in areas under control have clearly demonstrated some successes, highlighting advances in the application of new or expanded sets of tools to address human helminthiases. Anthelmintics are in general safe, can be successfully delivered through mass drug administration (MDA), and are being donated or their prices have fallen sharply, and there are promising advances in vaccine development. Also, high-risk populations including pregnant women and young children can be treated in the case of several infections (e.g. soil-transmitted helminthiases (STHs)), and some studies now indicate that treatment with praziquantel (PZQ) for schistosomiasis in small children and pregnant women is acceptable. There are new geostatistical tools for the mapping of infection distribution, and community-directed interventions have enabled the delivery of rapid-impact intervention packages more efficiently, reaching wider populations and covering a wider range of infections. One major obstacle for many research studies is the problem that most of the human helminths cannot be cultured in vitro or maintained in small animal models throughout their full life-cycles. However, enough is known about their biology from indirect studies to identify novel targets for drugs and vaccines, which in the long run may improve the tools available for prevention and control of helminth infections. The major advances in the different areas of helminth research are summarized below.

4.1 Advances in interventions and their monitoring and evaluation

For the control of onchocerciasis and lymphatic filariasis (LF), intervention is largely dependent on MDA in which communities at risk are treated in order to reduce morbidity and parasite transmission. In the case of LF, topical treatment of individuals with affected limbs or other organs with antimicrobial washing may be used as an adjunct treatment to reduce morbidity (95). The mass chemotherapy programmes aim to achieve a high level of coverage (65%–90%) of the eligible population. For onchocerciasis, the only drug available for safe and mass treatment remains ivermectin (IVM). For LF, mass chemotherapy is based on diethylcarbamazine (DEC) plus albendazole (ABZ) or DEC alone, except in Sub-Saharan Africa (SSA) where IVM plus ABZ is used because of contraindications for DEC in patients heavily infected with *O. volvulus*. Currently, tens of millions of people in hyper- and mesoendemic areas are under annual or semi-annual treatment for onchocerciasis, while hundreds of millions of people are under annual treatment for LF. A major problem is that the use of IVM in areas where loiasis (caused by *Loa loa*) is co-endemic can be contra-indicated due to rare, yet severe adverse events (SAEs), including fatalities (*96*).

Ivermectin is microfilaricidal and also suppresses adult worm fecundity (production of new microfilariae (mf)) for several months in onchocerciasis (*97*) and LF (*98*). DEC also is microfilaricidal, suppresses adult worm reproduction for several months, and kills a proportion of adult lymphatic filariae. ABZ too appears to contribute to the suppression of adult worm reproduction (*99*); it also has significant effects on most STHs, producing ancillary benefits among those treated.

Mass treatment programmes for onchocerciasis and LF are dramatically reducing morbidity and transmission. In some foci of the Americas, Mali, Senegal and Nigeria (Kaduna), there has been encouraging evidence that the elimination of onchocerciasis may be possible through MDA with IVM, when high levels of therapeutic and geographic coverage over many years have been achieved (14 years in Mali and Senegal) (*57*). Similarly, encouraging results have been achieved from efforts to eliminate LF in some parts of the world (e.g. Egypt) (*53*).

MDA programmes for STHs are most often directed at school-age children as they are the population group most at risk of acquiring heavy infection and developing associated morbidity, and most accessible for intervention through school-based programmes. However, some mass chemotherapy programmes are directed at whole communities in highly endemic areas.

The scale of MDA interventions for STHs has increased significantly in recent years (e.g. PPC; DtW, see Table 1, page 7). The focus of these interventions is to achieve long-term reductions in infection prevalence and intensity, and consequently of associated morbidity, rather than to eliminate the reservoir of infection. The aims of STH programmes are closely related to those of poverty reduction, and improvements in education and sanitation. However, awareness has recently increased that none of the anthelmintics used for STH, when used as monotherapy, is highly efficacious against hookworms and whipworms, although activity against *A. lumbricoides* may be high. Recently, the genetic polymorphisms in β-tubulin, which cause benzimidazole (BZ) resistance in livestock parasites, have been found in *T. trichiura* and *N. americanus*, and DNA assays to detect the occurrence of these single nucleotide polymorphisms (SNPs) have been developed so that resistance-associated SNPs can be monitored in stool samples of STH eggs (*100*).

Interventions for the control of schistosome infections involve MDA and/or chemotherapy of individuals, as well as improved sanitation, environmental modifications to reduce exposure to the snail intermediate hosts and to shed cercariae, and education to reduce unsafe water contact. An important recent advance in the control of schistosome infections has been the demonstration that artemisinin-based compounds (e.g. artemether) can be highly effective against schistosomes, particularly immature schistosomes which are relatively refractory to PZQ (*101*). The artemisinins could prove useful should PZQ resistance become a problem (*102*), however, only in special settings of known exposure. As artemisinins kill mainly immature worms and it is hard to know when someone has immature worms in truly endemic settings, this makes it difficult to know when to treat, making it difficult to use these drugs in anti-schistosomiasis MDA. Moreover, the artemisinins are currently critically important for antimalarial chemotherapy (in the light of resistance to most other antimalarials). Therefore, PZQ is virtually the only anti-schistosome medication used in MDA programmes.

Although rodents can harbour S. mansoni, S. haematobium does not have non-human reservoirs, which facilitates control. Occasional infections with S. bovis in situations promoting very close proximity between humans and cattle have been reported (*103*). S. japonicum, in contrast, is a zoonosis and there have been important recent advances in identifying which animal species play an important role in transmission among themselves and to humans in the People's Republic of China (PRC) (*104, 105*) and the Philippines (*106, 107*). The Disease Reference Group 6 (DRG6) report discusses how the contribution of different animal species to infection in humans may vary in endemic areas – the relative contribution of mammals such as cattle, water buffalo, wild rodents, dogs and cats in the transmission of S. japonicum to humans has been shown to vary significantly in different geographic and epidemiologic settings. Recent reports from the Philippines show quite conclusively that water buffalo are also the main non-human reservoir, as in marshland areas of the PRC (*108*).

Schistosomiasis control programmes under the umbrella of Schistosomiasis Control Initiative (SCI) activities are making progress towards the reduction of prevalence and intensity of infection and morbidity in sub-Saharan Africa (SSA), with encouraging results from Mali (*109*), Burkina Faso (*110*), and Uganda (*111*). In the latter, reductions in incidence have also been demonstrated, bringing benefits not only to those treated but also to those untreated members of the communities (*59*). Spatial mapping of schistosomiasis has been significantly advanced in both West (*112*) and East Africa (*113*). Operations research has highlighted the potential of Lot Quality Assurance (LQA) sampling for identifying high risk communities for S. mansoni (*114*).

Recognition that liver fluke infection can be a significant cause of hepatic cancer is an important scientific advance in this field (*115*). A more aggressive education programme in South-East Asia could produce long-term reductions in liver fluke induced morbidity. This will involve greater recognition of the importance of these infections and greater efforts to prevent infection. Prevention and control of human liver fluke infections can be facilitated by treatment of human and animal reservoirs with PZQ (to reduce egg shedding), improved sanitation (to prevent eggs from reaching water sources), and health education (to discourage consumption of raw fish and improve sanitary and food hygiene practices). Food-borne trematodes including the liver flukes mentioned above are discussed in detail in the DRG6 report. The report also refers to the carcinogenic effect of *Op. viverrini* – long-term infection can cause cholangiocarcinoma. The report also mentions PZQ as exhibiting a safe broad spectrum of activity against trematodes as well as having an excellent safety profile, making it the drug of choice for liver flukes among others.

Control of *Taenia* spp. infections has greatly improved with the introduction of concomitant porcine chemotherapy using oxfendazole, and the development of TSOL18 as a highly effective porcine vaccine (*116*). Proof of concept of the feasibility of actively eliminating *T. solium* transmission has also been provided recently in a wide endemic area of Peru and in Cameroon (*117, 118*). The DRG6 report refers to the WHO's inclusion of cysticercosis/taeniasis in its Global Plan to combat Neglected Tropical Diseases 2008–2009, using new initiatives addressing integrated control of zoonotic diseases and assessing the burden of food-borne disease. The report discusses cysticercosis/taeniasis in detail and provides evidence from randomized community trials on the effectiveness of strategies to control cysticercosis through combined mass human and pig chemotherapy. The evidence supported some reduction of prevalence and incidence of porcine cysticercosis in the intervention villages compared to the controls. Further discussion on cysticercosis/taeniasis is also provided in the DRG6 report.

4.2 Analysis of the tools for control interventions

4.2.1 Anthelmintic pharmaceuticals and their modalities of delivery

Most helminth control programmes today concentrate heavily on treatment and have achieved good results in terms of decreasing the intensity and prevalence of infection in some endemic areas (*50–52*). One reason for this heavy reliance on anthelmintics is because the cost of anthelmintics is relatively modest (*2*). Among the limitations of these programmes is that they do not incorporate environmental components such as improvement of sanitation and drainage, access to clean water, adequate sewage disposal, access to health services for monitoring and diagnosis, housing that limits access of vectors, and health education for achieving integrated and sustainable control (*52, 61*). Controversy remains regarding the optimal control strategy: mass treatment vs. focus on specific risk groups, such as school-aged children and at-risk occupational groups (*119–121*), and how these strategies impact on infection, morbidity, and compliance of the participating population. There is a need for research to evaluate factors that affect compliance, including sociological and behavioural factors (*51, 122–125*). The efficacy of many MDA programmes appears to be lower than originally envisaged and, depending on the initial level of endemicity (typically measured in terms of infection prevalence) and the life-span of the parasites, it may be necessary to extend the duration of such programmes for longer than originally envisioned. This can lead to treatment coverage declining ('community fatigue'), political will and financial support wavering ('donor fatigue'), and risk the development of drug resistance (126). What is typically seen is a pattern of rapid decline in infection intensity levels, followed by declines in infection prevalence in the first few years after commencement of the MDA programme (when the proportional gains are largest). However, after these initial gains, prevalence and intensity may enter a period during which they remain at a low level, but do not proceed to zero, as predicted at the beginning of the MDA programme. Poor compliance can be a factor in the persistence of infection, and often treatment coverage decreases as the programme advances. Often antiparasitic drugs also require the participation of a competent host immune system to be fully effective. Heterologous host responses and diversity in the parasite population may contribute to persistence of infection in some control programmes. It is important to look at individual responses to treatment (variance in the response) and not only at averages to understand why infection persists in some individuals/communities; it is in the outlier responses that explanations for suboptimal outcomes, including the possibility of drug resistance, can be found (127).

Other explanations for suboptimal outcomes in MDA programmes also need to be considered. These include the quality of the drug (pharmaceutical factors), the possibility that some individuals may have compromised immunity or altered pharmacokinetic handling of the drugs (patient factors), migration of previously untreated people (and/or movement of infected vectors) into the control programme area (which results in an influx of parasites), or that the parasites are not responding to treatment as predicted from previous clinical and field trials (parasite factors). This latter may be seen when drug resistance is selected or a particular parasite population is less responsive than populations seen elsewhere (tolerance or natural resistance in parasite sub-populations). Where possible, a variety of alternative explanations should be examined and some, such as therapeutic coverage, intensity of ongoing transmission, and response to treatment/possible resistance should be monitored on an ongoing basis. While suboptimal drug quality can lead to unsatisfactory results, this is more likely to occur when the anthelmintic is sourced from unregulated manufacturers and should not occur when the drug is supplied by the originator pharmaceutical company, as occurs in the case of all of the donated pharmaceuticals mentioned below. While patient factors such as compromised immunity, atypical pharmacokinetic handling of the drug, or migration of a small number of untreated individuals with high infection levels may occur, the small number of such subjects makes this an unlikely explanation for suboptimal programmatic results. Provided that, in monitoring and evaluation studies, the sample sizes are large enough, the population groups followed have been adequately chosen according to the infection biology and epidemiology (*128*), and other factors (e.g. drug source) are adequately controlled, other explanations such as inadequate coverage, poor compliance, parasite influx from surrounding areas not under MDA, and drug resistance development must be considered and carefully evaluated to assess their relative contributions to sub-optimal responses to MDA. Provided adequate treatment records are kept and maintained, it should be possible to evaluate treatment coverage. However, other methods may be necessary to assess fully an individual's compliance (*129*). High levels of parasite influx into areas under control are possible if migration of infected, untreated people occurs on a large scale (e.g. relocation of populations, forced displacement under conflict or natural disasters); it may also occur through movement/transport of infected vectors/intermediate hosts. Under normal circumstances and in large areas under control this becomes more unlikely since surrounding areas are also likely to be under MDA (and not have high levels of endemicity). Possible decreases in drug efficacy and emerging drug resistance are at present hard to assess due to a paucity of standardized methods for the assessment of drug efficacy in human helminthiases and the lack of drug resistance markers, and so these factors are frequently ignored. There is also the perception that drug resistance fears may compromise the commitment of populations, donors and governments and damage control programmes, not recognizing that lack of prompt and decisive action may have far more serious long-term consequences.

It should be recognized that drug treatment regimes are often not optimized for treatment of human populations in helminth control strategies (*130*), let alone in integrated programmes for multiple neglected tropical disease (NTD) control, in which drug combinations need to be co-administered simultaneously or in staggered protocols. Very often dose rates have been extrapolated from veterinary studies and treatment regimes designed to reduce the need for repeat treatment (*130*). From the point of view of large-scale and community-directed anthelmintic delivery, these may be important and practical considerations. However, as discussed above, often drug efficacy in operational settings is lower than desirable. This can have the consequences that the level of control/transmission interruption that is achieved is sub-optimal, and may increase selection pressure for drug resistance to develop. A related problem is the difficulty in accurately assessing the efficacy of anthelmintics. Reliable biomarkers could assist the assessment of efficacy and this constitutes an important research challenge that is discussed below (see section 4.4).

For all of the human helminthiases, there is a paucity of pharmaceuticals available for the reasons given in section 1.1. This is of concern in view of the increasing deployment of large-scale MDA programmes using only one or a few drugs, with none in reserve, and the increased possibility of development of drug resistance. There is a critical need for new anthelmintic drugs to be specifically developed for human use (*130*).

Filarial infections: Currently, tens of millions of people in hyper- and mesoendemic areas are under annual or semi-annual treatment for onchocerciasis, while hundreds of millions of people are under annual treatment for LF. There is a need to develop and register a paediatric formulation of IVM for onchocerciasis and LF control. Such a formulation would allow community coverage to be increased in MDA programmes. In some areas, filarial infections and transmission still persist despite many years of MDA. In some cases, this could be attributed to less than optimal treatment coverage leading to ongoing transmission, human host factors relating to treatment adherence, failure to include vector control in addition to drug treatment (*63, 131*), and to other factors not yet fully understood. The latter may include parasite genetic factors such as heterogeneity in drug susceptibility, and selection pressure from repeated treatment resulting in development of drug resistance. Research challenges therefore include the implementation of studies designed to understand the relative contributions of treatment coverage, compliance patterns, intensity of infection, intensity of transmission, and parasite genetics/drug resistance to the ability of individual hosts and their parasites to respond to treatment.

Regarding the frequency of treatment, annual treatment, although effective in reducing microfilarial load and morbidity, may not be optimal for interruption of *O. volvulus* transmission, nor reduce selection for IVM resistance compared with semi-annual treatment. More frequent treatment further reduces microfilarial load and transmission to vectors, and may therefore reduce the fitness advantage conferred to female worms that return more rapidly to fertility after IVM treatment. However, the logistic burden of providing semi-annual treatment and its possible effect on increasing the rate of selection for resistance (the simple argument that more frequent treatment would increase the pressure to select for resistant worms) may make annual IVM treatment a better option. These are important research questions that have not yet been addressed. They need to be addressed at first in a treatment setting where no or few rounds of IVM treatment have been dispensed (no existing selection towards drug resistance), and secondly, in a situation where there have been many rounds of IVM treatment and there is evidence of selection for sub-optimal responses.

Moxidectin is under development for use in humans for onchocerciasis treatment. However, further research is needed to ascertain if it has advantages relative to IVM for onchocerciasis control. The development of IVM resistance may compromise moxidectin as both drugs appear to share (in veterinary nematodes) some resistance mechanisms. This issue will require research should moxidectin be employed for human onchocerciasis. Another potential new drug development strategy is the possible use of antibiotics to target the *Wolbachia* endosymbionts in *O. volvulus* and lymphatic filariae. However, at present the recommended antibiotic, doxycycline, seems unlikely to be suitable for large-scale mass chemotherapy due to the long course of daily treatment required to obtain desirable effects (six weeks) and the inability to use the drug in young children and pregnant women. Field trials have been conducted to test the feasibility of administering doxycycline via community distributors with good coverage and compliance in areas endemic for both onchocerciasis and loiasis (*132*). Given that *L. loa* is one of the filarial parasites with no *Wolbachia*, this is a promising result that would allow treatment in those co-endemic areas where IVM cannot be used (those in which the prevalence of loiasis is greater than 20%). Research programmes to identify alternative antibiotics that might be as effective but require shorter courses of treatment are under way (*94*). Should moxidectin prove to have advantages for onchocerciasis control, consideration should be given for its use against lymphatic filariae. In veterinary use, long-acting formulations of moxidectin have been developed with significant benefits against filarial parasites. Such long-acting formulations could be useful if current development efforts with moxidectin prove successful. Continued efforts are required to develop more effective antifilarial anthelmintics, and particularly to find drugs with macrofilaricidal activity. Moreover, leads from the veterinary field, such as emodepside and monepantel, should be assessed for activity against human filariae and STHs.

The dose rates of IVM and ABZ used for LF control may be sub-optimal (*130*). Optimization of dosing for these drugs will require additional research. For logistic reasons, yearly treatments have been adopted for LF elimination. The effect of more frequent treatment (6–9 months) with either DEC, DEC + ABZ or IVM + ABZ on decreasing transmission, thereby shortening the time required to achieve elimination, should be studied. In addition, the advantages of more frequent treatment with ABZ (and IVM) on reducing morbidity due to STHs as a collateral benefit of treatment for LF may be greater than achieved with annual treatment.

As mentioned, the use of IVM in loiasis co-endemic areas where some individuals exhibit high-level microfilaraemia can be contra-indicated due to rare SAEs, including death. The occurrence of SAEs following IVM treatment in some (but not all) subjects with high burdens of *L. loa* requires urgent research. The occurrences of SAEs seem to be largely confined to Cameroon, Democratic Republic of Congo, and Sudan, even though *L. loa* has a wider distribution. Certainly, high burdens of *L. loa* are a predisposing condition, but may not be the only factor predisposing to SAEs. Recent research (*133*) suggests that a genetic polymorphism in ABC transporters at the blood-brain barrier may also be a predisposing factor. This problem requires urgent attention as such SAEs can be fatal, and their occurrence is critically limiting efforts to control onchocerciasis and LF in regions of Africa.

Soil-transmitted helminthiases: The efficacy of anthelmintics against hookworms and *T. trichiura* is less than satisfactory (*130*). Research is required to optimize dose rates of existing drugs for these STHs. In addition, the evidence that part of the cause of the low/variable efficacy of ABZ (or mebendazole (MBZ)) in *T. trichiura* and *N. americanus* may be due to BZ-resistant genotypes of these parasites occurring in some populations (*134*) needs urgent investigation, as a lack of understanding on this issue may jeopardize the sustainability of control efforts against STHs. Another research need is that of assessing the effectiveness of new anthelmintics, such as nitazoxanide and tribendimidine for MDA of STHs, and combination therapy (discussed below).

Schistosomiasis and other trematode infections: The development and thorough evaluation of a paediatric formulation of PZQ (such as PZQ syrup) would allow greater population coverage in MDA programmes against schistosomiasis. In some parts of the PRC and the Philippines, where bovines can act as a reservoir for *S. japonicum* (*104, 108*), treatment or vaccination of this reservoir host has the potential to improve the efficacy of control programmes. An anti-schistosome fecundity vaccine with an efficacy of 50%–90% is currently being tested (*135*). While PZQ is usually highly effective against adult schistosomes, its efficacy may be poor against immature infections (*136*). As noted above, the artemisinins appear to have good activity against immature stages. Currently however, there is a reluctance to develop artemisinins for anti-schistosome chemotherapy because of the key role the drugs play in antimalarial chemotherapy and concern that overuse of the drugs could select for strains of malaria parasites resistant to artemisinins. Nevertheless, experimental studies on the use of artemisinins, alone or in combination with PZQ, may be appropriate. Artemisinins may represent an arm of improved chemotherapy for schistosomiasis, and as a possible means of reducing selection for potential PZQ resistance, but only in special circumstances, due to their limited impact on adult worms. They might work well in some very high transmission places but only where there are likely to be a lot of immature worms in those being treated.

Taeniasis and other cestode infections: Prevention and control of *Taenia* spp. infections should involve enhanced sanitation and health education (to improve sanitary practices). These measures by themselves, however, are unlikely to be sufficient for control, and thus interventions including human mass chemotherapy, porcine chemotherapy or porcine immunization are required. Chemotherapy with niclosamide has limited efficacy, and the use of PZQ carries the theoretical risk of triggering seizures in asymptomatic individuals with neurocysticercosis (NCC). Mass vaccination of pigs with the TSOL18 vaccine, which can be close to 100% effective, is a promising intervention (*137*).

4.2.2 Efficacy of anthelmintics

In the case of filarial parasites, anthelmintics only kill some (DEC in LF) or very few (IVM, ABZ) adult worms, but do temporarily (from several to many weeks) sterilize the adult worms and kill mf. Thus, to ascertain phenotypic effects of anthelmintics on filariae requires assessment of pre- and post-treatment microfilarial counts in blood (LF) or skin (onchocerciasis) at different times and/or assessment of reproductive status in the female worms (embryograms in the case of *O. volvulus* obtained from excised nodules). In the case of STHs, anthelmintic treatment is targeted to kill the mature stages of the helminth but, as it is difficult to assess killing of the adult worms in humans directly, efficacy has to be assessed in terms of faecal egg count reductions or cure rates.

The efficacy of most of the existing anthelmintics against STHs is at best mediocre (even in the absence of any drug resistance). Keiser & Utzinger (*138*) conducted a meta-analysis of the efficacy of ABZ, MBZ and pyrantel pamoate, while Stepek et al. (*139*) provided additional data on the efficacy of IVM and levamisole against STHs (Table 2). As can be seen from these analyses, the efficacy of single dose anthelmintic therapy against STHs is very variable and, with the possible exception of the efficacy of most anthelmintics against *A. lumbricoides*, is unsatisfactory. In many cases, the dose rates of the anthelmintic or dose regimen may not be optimal (*130*). However, other factors, possibly including a level of innate anthelmintic tolerance (see below) may also contribute to low efficacy in some instances. New anthelmintics for STHs, such as tribendimidine (which shares a mechanism of action with levamisole and pyrantel) (*140*), and nitazoxanide do not have superior efficacies compared with those commonly used and shown in Table 2 (*130*).

4.2.3 Anthelmintic resistance

With the increasing reliance of large-scale MDA programmes on single dose therapy with partially effective drugs, and the fact that the same few anthelmintics have been in use for 20 to 30 years, the risk of drug resistance developing has increased. With all of the anthelmintics there is a need to develop sensitive molecular markers to monitor for resistance. In the development of these markers it will be necessary to conduct studies in which the clinical and parasitological responses to treatment are measured at the same time as the frequency of resistance genotypes is assessed. This would establish the association between the markers and the biological outcome of the treatment. In addition to research to find optimal molecular markers for resistance, the population structure of different parasites will need to be determined in order to assess the likely rate of spread of resistant populations and the possibility of recrudescence of infection in areas where infection is initially eliminated.

Table 2
Mean cure rates (%) of anthelmintics against intestinal nematodes (95% confidence interval)

Drug	Dose	Necator americanus; Ancylostoma duodenale* (hookworms)	Trichuris trichiura (whipworm)	Ascaris lumbricoides (roundworm)	Enterobius vermicularis (pinworm)	Strongyloides stercoralis (threadworm)
Albendazole (ABZ)	400 mg	72 (59–81)	28 (13–39)	88 (79–93)	40–100[†]	17–95[†]
Mebendazole (MBZ)	500 mg	15 (1–27)	36 (16–51)	95 (91–97)	96[†]	44[†]
Ivermectin (IVM)	200 µg/kg	0–20[†]	11–80[†]	50–75[†]	61–94[†]	83–100[†]
Pyrantel	10 mg/kg	31 (19–42)	0–56[†]	88 (79–93)	>90[†]	–
Levamisole	2.5 mg/kg	66–100[†]	16–18[†]	86–100[†]	–	–

Adapted from Keiser & Utzinger (138) and [†]Stepek et al. (139).
* An. duodenale is usually much more susceptible to most anthelmintics than N. americanus.
[†] Indicates range or single value.

In nematode parasites of farmed ruminants and domestic animals, there is a serious problem of anthelmintic resistance to all of the anthelmintics which are currently used in humans (except DEC which is rarely used in livestock and companion animals) (*141*). In parasites of veterinary importance, phenotypic evidence of resistance often goes undetected, as it has been estimated that the level of resistance would have to reach at least 25% before it can be detected with conventional egg count reduction assays for assessing anthelmintic efficacy (*142*). This same insensitivity also exists with assessment of efficacy in human STHs. A limited number of efficacy studies published on hookworms in humans raise the possibility of resistance, but are inconclusive. The study of De Clercq et al. (*143*) in Mali on *N. americanus* was suggestive that resistance against MBZ had developed (clearance rate of 22.9%, hookworm egg reduction rate (ERR) of 6.5%, ED50 of 0.117 instead of 0.069). However, when these authors compared the efficacy of pyrantel, ABZ and MBZ in the same localities, they fell short of providing conclusive evidence of resistance against MBZ (*144*). Reynoldson et al. (*145*) suggested that the *An. duodenale* found in a region of Australia was resistant to pyrantel, but the results were based on only 15 individuals. On Pemba Island, Zanzibar, the efficacy of MBZ against hookworms in schoolchildren appeared to have fallen over a period of five years, during which time the children were regularly treated with MBZ (ERR fell from 82.4% to 52.1%). This suggested the possibility of MBZ resistance emerging in hookworms (*146*). Recently, a single dose of MBZ was found to have disappointing efficacy (ERR of 31%) against hookworm infections in Vietnam (*147*), although single dose and repeated ABZ treatment achieved higher efficacy (88% and 75%, respectively). Because the efficacy of anthelmintics against hookworms is normally only moderate, it is hard to draw definitive conclusions from these studies. The presence of genetic changes in polymorphic loci associated with BZ resistance in veterinary nematodes would at least provide evidence that resistance has the potential to occur. Albonico et al. (*148*) examined the β-tubulin cDNA sequence of one *An. duodenale* and 71 *N. americanus* worms isolated from stool samples following MBZ treatment (i.e. worms expelled by the treatment and thus likely to be susceptible to the anthelmintic) in the efficacy study on Pemba Island mentioned above. Schwenkenbecher et al. (*149*) re-examined DNA samples extracted by Albonico et al. (*148*) and found a frequency of alleles associated with BZ susceptibility of almost 100% (the highest frequency of resistance alleles being 0.0046 for the resistance codon at position 167 of the β-tubulin gene). Diawara (*134*) also examined nine of the same Pemba samples by pyrosequencing, and confirmed the absence of the resistant codon at position 200. In contrast, when 20 pools of eggs from subjects in Haiti who had been under MBZ treatment for many years were examined (*100*), significant levels of putative resistance alleles were observed. Diawara et al. (*134*) developed genotyping assays for β-tubulin in *A. lumbricoides* and *T. trichiura* and found that *T. trichiura* worms from people in Panama, Haiti, and Kenya contained resistance-associated alleles. The occurrence of resistance-associated β-tubulin alleles in *T. trichiura* may explain why BZ anthelmintics are less effective against this species and indicates that ABZ/MBZ resistance in *T. trichiura* might be possible.

An important drug used against LF is DEC. However, neither its mechanism of action nor any possible resistance mechanisms are known, nor is there a test for possible DEC resistance. There are, however, periodic reports of unexpectedly poor clinical responses to DEC. Eberhard et al. (*150, 151*) reported persistence of LF microfilaraemia in Haiti after DEC treatment, and non-susceptibility in some Haitian *W. bancrofti* individual worms. More recently, Dixit et al. (*152*) reported a sharp decline in all therapeutic indices with the microfilarial count returning to pre-treatment levels by the 4th year of single annual DEC therapy. Even after 20 years of DEC, LF microfilaraemia may persist, particularly in the absence of concomitant vector control (*63, 131*). It is not known whether these and other reports of unsatisfactory response to MDA with DEC could, in part, be due to DEC resistance. MDA for LF is usually undertaken with combination DEC+ABZ or IVM+ABZ therapy. The genetic polymorphism in the β-tubulin gene, responsible for most ABZ/MBZ resistance in nematode parasites of farmed animals, occurs in *W. bancrofti* (*153*). A genetic polymorphism has also been found in *O. volvulus* β-tubulin (*154–156*), with 'resistance' allele frequencies increasing with the number of treatment rounds, suggesting that IVM exerts selective pressure on β-tubulin. Thus in areas where MDA with IVM+ABZ combination is implemented, there could be greater selection for ABZ resistance, via genetic selection on β-tubulin, than in areas where IVM is not used in combination with ABZ.

There is evidence that IVM resistance may be occurring in *O. volvulus* in some communities in Ghana that have been subjected to 12–17 rounds of IVM treatment with moderate to good levels of IVM coverage. This resistance is manifested as a greater ability of the adult female worms to recommence reproduction sooner after IVM treatment than had been observed previously. In addition, the persistence of *O. volvulus* mf in the skin after several treatments with this drug has been documented (*157–159*). Evidence to support drug resistance includes genetic selection by IVM on the genome of *O. volvulus* (*154–156, 160–165*). It had been suggested (*166*) that the sub-optimal rapid repopulation of skin mf in the three communities in Ghana studied by Osei-Atweneboana et al. (*159*) could be explained by new infections rather than IVM resistance, but examination of the age structure of adult female worms extracted at nodulectomy showed a scarcity of young worms. Similarly, embryograms of the adult female worms from the three communities showed no evidence of a skewed age structure towards younger worms, thus indicating that the rapid repopulation of the skin by mf was unlikely to be accounted for by a high level of new infections. A similar conclusion was reached by Churcher et al. (*127*).

However, there is a need to conduct transmission studies in the areas where suboptimal responses have been documented to further investigate the transmission dynamics in such communities. There is also a need to develop molecular markers for IVM resistance in *O. volvulus* and to use such markers to monitor, on an ongoing basis, for possible IVM resistance in areas under MDA with IVM. Continuous surveillance is critically important for treatment and prevention of recrudescence or reintroduction of helminth infections (*122*).

4.2.4 Combinations of anthelmintics

There are two reasons for considering the use of combination anthelmintics: firstly, to increase the spectrum, effectiveness and convenience of drug administration, and secondly, to slow the development of resistance. In the first instance two different anthelmintics might be given in order to integrate control programmes, e.g. schistosomiasis control with that of STH in schoolchildren, with PZQ and ABZ, in which each anthelmintic acts independently and targets different parasites. In the second instance, the anthelmintics may be given together (as separate medications or as a co-formulation) in order to increase the effectiveness of the drug treatment. Examples of this may be the co-administration of ABZ with DEC (or IVM) for LF. In this circumstance the DEC (or IVM) exhibits microfilaricidal activity, has some limited adulticidal activity (in the case of DEC), and causes a temporary inhibition of reproduction by the adult parasites (IVM and DEC), while the ABZ extends the duration of inhibition of reproduction and exerts activity against some STHs as a collateral benefit. These extensions of the spectrum or effectiveness of chemotherapy may be desirable in their own right. However, in addition to these possible benefits, combination chemotherapy has appeal as a means of reducing selection of drug resistance.

Antimalarial drug resistance is a major public health problem which hinders the control of malaria. Drug combinations, rather than monotherapy, are now seen to be the best solution for treating malaria, and artemisinin-based drug combinations are highly effective and recommended by the WHO (see report by the Disease Reference Group on Malaria, DRG1). The use of combinations to delay the development of anthelmintic resistance needs to be examined carefully so that appropriate combinations are used and optimized for this purpose. In the treatment of veterinary parasites, the use of anthelmintic combinations to slow the development of resistance has been promoted in Australia (*167*) and New Zealand (*168*) but remains controversial (*169, 170*). Much of the underlying science is based on studies with insecticides; some modelling studies have suggested that using combinations of insecticides will be better than using them sequentially or in rotation (*171–174*) while results from others have concluded that combinations probably offer few advantages in slowing the development of resistance and may even be worse than single-pesticide strategies under some conditions (*175*, *176*). However, the output from modelling studies will depend very much on the underlying assumptions that are made and so it is helpful to examine under which conditions combinations are likely to reduce the rate of selection for drug resistance. A number of conditions will impact whether combination chemotherapy, as opposed to monotherapy, should be effective in slowing the development of resistance. Combinations will be most beneficial when: 1) resistance mechanisms to the different anthelmintics in the combination are under independent genetic control, i.e. do not share common mechanisms of resistance/resistance genes; 2) the genes for resistance are functionally recessive at the dose rates to be used; 3) such genes are rare and the efficacy of each of the component compounds against the susceptible genotypes approaches 100%; 4) a proportion of the population is not exposed to treatment, i.e. some refugia exist; and 5) the compounds used have similar persistence (*171–173*, *175*). In these circumstances, anthelmintic combinations are likely to be beneficial in reducing the rate of selection for anthelmintic resistance.

At the current time, the anthelmintic armamentarium is unsatisfactory; for example, anthelmintics from different chemical classes may share similar resistance mechanisms and select on the same genes. There is a considerable literature indicating that ABC transporters are involved in IVM resistance (*177*, *178*). However, BZ anthelmintics such as ABZ and MBZ also appear to select on some ABC transporter genes (*179*, *180*). Furthermore, changes in the isotype β-tubulin gene are known to cause BZ resistance (*181*) while IVM also selects on the isotype 1 β-tubulin gene of some nematode parasites (*154*, *182*). Thus, a combination of ABZ and IVM may be useful in terms of broadening the spectrum/efficacy of the combination, compared with each anthelmintic individually, but it may not reduce the rate of selection for resistance to one or both components of the combination. While there is no evidence that BZ resistance causes cross-resistance to IVM, there is now some evidence that selection with IVM can select for BZ resistance (*183*). The other factor that hampers the use of anthelmintic combinations for human helminth infections, in terms of delaying selection for resistance, is that the efficacy of anthelmintics against human helminths is at best mediocre and is usually less than 100%. Further, there is some evidence, based on genotypic analysis, that mutations that normally result in BZ resistance are quite common in populations of *T. trichiura* (*134*). Thus, in the case of this parasite, little benefit in terms of protecting against selection of resistance using combinations that include ABZ may accrue. These examples point to the importance of assessing any proposed combination against the five criteria outlined in the previous paragraph before using such a combination as a means of delaying the selection for resistance. Nevertheless, there will be a role for combinations to expand spectrum or efficacy, as well as to provide increased convenience for mass administration programmes. However, more attention should be given to how well a proposed combination meets the criteria outlined above before the use of combinations (either two anthelmintics in the same formulation, or two anthelmintics in separate formulations given at the same time) is implemented.

In addition, pharmacokinetic and pharmacodynamic interactions of anthelmintics are poorly studied in humans. Some anthelmintics, such as IVM, are very potent ligands for some ABC transporters (*178*) and may alter the pharmacokinetics of the partner drug, in both the host and parasite, if they are substrates for the same ABC transporters, and thus may potentially increase toxicity to the host (undesirable) or to the parasite (desirable). There is evidence of complex interactions in vivo of levamisole and both IVM and ABZ sulfoxide (its active metabolite). Thus combination chemotherapy needs to be considered carefully and further research should be conducted before such combinations are deployed on a large scale (*184*).

4.2.5 Vector control

Vector control has been successful for onchocerciasis (*185*), schistosomiasis in PRC (*186*), and more locally in some LF foci, e.g. in Zanzibar (*187*) and India (*188*). In the case of onchocerciasis, vector control was widely used with considerable success in the early days of the Onchocerciasis Control Programme (OCP) in West Africa. However, its widespread use proved expensive, had some adverse environmental consequences, and led to insecticide resistance, which required careful monitoring and control, with the introduction and rotation of other insecticides (*189*). Widespread vector control has been abandoned, but can still be helpful in the control of onchocerciasis in limited foci, and the African Programme for Onchocerciasis Control (APOC) continues to conduct selective vector elimination programmes (e.g. the eradication of the (endemic) Bioko form of *Simulium yahense* in Bioko, and the elimination of *S. neavei* in Uganda). The addition of vector control may be particularly important where drug resistance is suspected, and also where elimination of the infection reservoir is being attempted. Many of the mosquito abatement programmes used in the control of malaria have had collateral impact on LF. As the vectors of LF tend to remain in the local environment, measures such as habitat spraying with insecticides (indoor residual spraying) and the use of insecticide treated bednets can help in the control of LF (and malaria), particularly in those areas (rural East Africa, West Africa, Papua New Guinea) where *Anopheles* mosquitoes transmit both *W. bancrofti* and *Plasmodium* spp. Further research on these measures, in combination with other interventions, is warranted. In areas where *Culex quinquefasciatus* is the main LF vector (this is the main vector of LF worldwide), adulticidal measures are less effective, and source reduction (e.g. use of expanded polystyrene beads in breeding sites such as pit-latrines and other receptacles) has been very effective for curbing transmission of LF in semi-urban/urban areas of Zanzibar (*187*) and southern India (*188*). Snail control for schistosomiasis has been helpful in the PRC (*186*) and Egypt, and in Japan it achieved elimination. However, potent molluscicides are sometimes general biocides and may need to be used with care under strict bio-surveillance for non-target organisms, and may be of most use in focal control and elimination situations.

4.2.6 Vaccines

Effective vaccines are, potentially, the most economical and efficient tools to control infectious diseases. The goal of MDA programmes is to alleviate infection and morbidity in the definitive host or to reduce transmission. A new strategy of positioning anti-helminth vaccines as adjunct and synergistic control measures provides a novel revitalizing concept in a field where control activities have remained exclusively focused on morbidity and/or transmission reduction using drug delivery. The development of anti-helminth vaccines that do not necessarily induce sterilizing immunity would reduce the likelihood of vaccinated individuals to develop severe infections and thus reduce the burden of disease throughout the world. It could be also argued that the success of control initiatives constitutes the justification needed for vaccine development, since an effective vaccine would add the necessary long-term perspective presently lacking in most of the control strategies. Not only would vaccine-linked chemotherapy reduce overall morbidity, but it would also reduce rates of parasite infection and re-infection. This in turn, would prolong the interval between repeated drug treatments and reduce the likelihood of drug resistance, thereby increasing the life-span of our current anthelmintic pharmacopoeia (*190*, *191*). There is also evidence that vaccination-induced immune responses are increased following anthelmintic chemotherapy, possibly because of reversal of immune suppression induced by the adult worms (*192*), or because of the release, and immunological presentation, of previously hidden helminth antigens following treatment (*135*, *193*). Importantly, the conceptual underpinning that a vaccine can be produced against helminth infections has been established and there is a need to further support activities to develop effective vaccines.

There have been some promising leads for the development of vaccines against human hookworm infections and against *O. volvulus* and schistosomiasis (*190*, *191*, *194*, *195*). However, other than the TSOL18 porcine vaccine for cysticercosis, there is a dearth of vaccines for prevention or control of human helminthiases. Although it is very expensive to develop a vaccine for use in humans, in view of the very high efficacy and safety of the TSOL18 vaccine in pigs and the very serious morbidity caused by NCC in humans, it would be desirable to assess the potential for using TSOL18 for prevention of *Taenia* infections in humans. The water buffalo trials mentioned earlier are another example of possible development of a veterinary vaccine that would lower transmission to humans.

Research to develop possible vaccines against helminth infections should be encouraged (*190, 191, 196, 197*). In the long term, vaccines should be the preferable means of prevention in the light of possible drug resistance development and the uncertainty as to whether chemotherapy-based programmes, which have to be repeated year after year, are sustainable or will be prone to the fatigue of donors, health agencies, and patients. Although it is unlikely that anti-helminthic vaccines will become 'magic bullets', they could be excellent adjunct measures when combined with other interventions for integrated helminth control.

4.3 Advances in tools for diagnosis of infection and surveillance of interventions

A number of significant considerations are resulting in advances in diagnostic technologies that are essential to the control of helminthiases. These include: 1) the convergence of epidemiological and laboratory approaches to develop tools optimal for control programmes, facilitated by the recognition that parasitological diagnosis at the individual level is not appropriate for implementing and monitoring such interventions (*198–200*); and 2) the application of modern laboratory techniques to diagnosis, exemplified by the use of polymerase chain reaction (PCR) (*53, 201*) and molecular techniques to produce parasite recombinant proteins as reagents for serodiagnostic tests (*202, 203*). Gaps in research related to diagnosis for epidemiology and surveillance are presented in section 8.2.

4.4 Analysis of the tools for diagnosis, monitoring and evaluation, and surveillance and their challenges

Techniques appropriate for diagnosis and surveillance of helminthiases are fundamental to overcoming many of the challenges to control of helminthiases. To address these challenges, it is necessary to understand the performance characteristics of currently available tools for diagnosis for each of the human helminth infections, and thereby identify critical gaps in diagnostic technology. Challenges include: quantifying intensity of infection; response to anthelmintic chemotherapy, including detection of anthelmintic resistance; disease mapping and surveillance; elimination; and the need to collect data amenable to use in mathematical modelling of infection. Infection intensity is defined here as the average number of parasites per host or of transmission stages (eggs, larvae, mf) per sampling unit (e.g. per gram of faeces, per volume of urine, per mg of skin, per ml of blood, depending on parasite species), taking into account both infected and uninfected hosts. Table 3 describes how the need for diagnostic assays changes according to the stage of the intervention.

Table 3
Monitoring and surveillance tools as control programmes advance

Helminthiasis	Stage of the control programme			References
	Early	Advanced	Final and end-point	
Onchocerciasis	Nodule palpation for detection of onchocercomata, skin-snipping for detection and counting of mf in skin snips	Skin snipping sensitivity decreases; DEC patch test; PCR-based monitoring of simuliid populations Ov-16 card test	Xenomonitoring via fly feeding/ recording microfilarial uptake. Serology in untreated children; PCR and DEC patch test; Ov-16 card test	(202, 204)
Lymphatic filariasis	Blood smears for detection and counting of mf in blood; circulating filarial antigen (CFA) for bancroftian filariasis. Rapid dipstick for detection of antibodies (Ab) in brugian filariasis	PCR-based assays for *W. bancrofti* and *B. malayi* in blood; PCR-based monitoring of mosquito populations	Monitoring infections in mosquitoes; anti-filarial Ab levels in children. Both serve as indicators of local transmission for making decisions about programme end-points	(203, 205, 206)
Soil-transmitted helminths	Quantitative egg counts using validated methodology (e.g. Kato-Katz (KK))	Infections become lighter and more difficult to detect; egg concentration techniques e.g. Flotac® likely to be required to detect light infections	Increasing proportion of unfertilized *Ascaris* eggs could indicate declining mating probability (unfertilized eggs often missed by KK). Need for highly sensitive diagnostic methods	(207)

continues

Table 3 continued

Helminthiasis	Stage of the control programme			References
	Early	Advanced	Final and end-point	
Intestinal schistosomiasis due to S. mansoni	As above	Need to validate PCR-based diagnostic assays in low-transmission areas	Elimination of infection reservoir rarely attempted	(208)
Intestinal schistosomiasis due to S. japonicum	Initial screening for antibodies in indirect haemagglutination assay (IHA); subsequent testing with KK of the seropositive individuals	Seroprevalence determined by IHA can be much higher than prevalence in stool-based PCR; hatching and KK tests	Develop new algorithms for treatment in low intensity areas; PCR may replace KK in such algorithms. Surveillance in snails; sentinel mice	(208–210)
Urinary schistosomiasis (S. haematobium)	Urine filtration for detection and counting of eggs	Need to improve urine circulating antigen test for use in low-transmission areas	Find and treat cases in both active surveillance and health-care settings	(208)

continues

Table 3 continued

Helminthiasis	Stage of the control programme			References
	Early	Advanced	Final and end-point	
Food-borne trematodiases	Detection of eggs in faeces (intestinal liver and lung flukes) and sputum (lung flukes) using KK or formalin-ethyl-acetate concentration. Species-specific diagnosis difficult due to similar egg morphology. Definite diagnosis may require adult worm examination following expulsion chemotherapy	Examination of multiple stool and sputum samples; use combination of diagnostic tests to enhance sensitivity. Flotac® in the process of validation. Immunodiagnostic tests under development. PCR-based methods to detect trematode DNA in stool or metacercariae in 2nd intermediate hosts (not yet available for routine use)	–	(33)
Cestode infections including taeniasis, cysticercosis	Microscopic examination of faeces to detect Taenia eggs (T. solium/T. saginata). Detection of tapeworm antigen in stools using ELISA copro-antigen detection (the latter not yet available for routine use)	Coproantigen detection to identify carriers and confirm post-treatment cure. Magnetic immuno-chromatographic tests (MICT) for detection of human antibodies to T. solium and NCC (under development)	–	(211, 212)

4.4.1 Diagnostics for filariases

Parasitological diagnosis: The filarial parasites (*O. volvulus*, *W. bancrofti* and *B. malayi*) are amenable to parasitological diagnosis by detection of microfilariae (mf). Microfilariae are found in the skin in *O. volvulus* and in the blood for the other two species. For lymphatic filariae, the timing of blood collection should coincide with the time of peak microfilaraemia, most often in the middle of the night, resulting in significant inconvenience. For *O. volvulus* infection, the collection and examination of skin snips is a well standardized, if sub-optimal, test; it lacks sensitivity in light infections, and may depend on the anatomic site from which the skin snips are taken, the number of snips taken, and the duration of snip incubation as well as composition of the incubation medium (*213*). This technique can only detect (by inference) the presence of fertile adult females and not early infection with young worms (pre-patent infection). The DEC patch test, where diethylcarbamazine is applied to a patch of skin, eliciting a so-called Mazzotti reaction (*214*), is a useful test for *O. volvulus* microfilarial prevalence. As the presence of heavy loads of *Loa loa* has been associated with rare SAEs in people being treated with IVM for onchocerciasis or LF (see above), the diagnosis of heavy *L. loa* infection can be of significant importance. *Loa loa* microfilaraemia can be detected in the blood during the day using one of several methods (thick smear, haemofiltration, etc). The presence of adult filarial worms can be detected by nodule palpation in *O. volvulus* infection, and by ultrasound examination of lymph nodes to detect worm nests in lymphatic filariasis. These adult worm detection methodologies have specific, albeit limited, uses (Table 4).

Antibody tests: Antibody tests have specific utility in the diagnosis of filarial infections, particularly in *O. volvulus* elimination. Using either a single *O. volvulus* recombinant protein or a pool of different recombinant proteins it is possible to screen sub-groups in a population, particularly children, for parasite-specific antibodies to these proteins, and to certify the interruption of transmission by establishing lack of antibody responsiveness (*204, 215–217*). Likewise, mapping of *L. loa* prevalence, in the context of possible IVM-induced SAEs, based on antibody response to a recombinant protein has been described (*218*).

For LF, sero-responsiveness to *B. malayi* adult worm antigens has been widely used in clinical diagnostic settings. When the antibody response to whole parasite antigen is measured, significant cross-reactivity with other nematode infections limits its applicability, and sero-reversion may be delayed. In the absence of a circulating antigen test for brugian filariasis (see below), a dipstick antibody test has been developed for diagnosis of *B. malayi* infection, based on antibody response to a recombinant *B. malayi* protein BmR1 (*219*).

Table 4
A Comparison of diagnostic tests for human onchocerciasis

Test	Specificity	Sensitivity	Interference by *O. ochengi*	Throughput	Cost	Application
Skin Snip	≤100%	Low	No	Low	Low	Field
Nodule Palpation	Moderate	Low	No	High	Low	Field
Snip PCR	≤100%	≤100%	No	Low	High	Lab
Scratch PCR	≤100%	≤100%	No	Low	High	Lab
DEC Patch	98%	36%–83%	No	Low	Low	Lab
Fly Dissection	Low	Low	Yes	Low	Moderate	Field
Fly pool PCR	High	High	No	High	Varies	Lab
Ab ELISA	≤100%	≤100%	No	High	Mod	Lab

Modified from Boatin et al. (*202*)

Antigen detection: A major advance in the diagnostic armamentarium for bancroftian filariasis is the development of antigen-capture assays enabling detection of circulating filarial antigen (CFA) of *W. bancrofti* (*220, 221*). This has enabled case-based diagnosis without the need for nocturnal blood collection, assessment of cure through clearance of antigenaemia (*222*), epidemiological mapping of endemicity (*223*), and is showing utility as a tool for elimination (*53*). No equivalent tests have been successfully developed for brugian filariasis, loiasis or onchocerciasis.

Molecular diagnosis: PCR-based tests have assumed a major place in the diagnostic arsenal for filariasis, particularly for assessment of infection in mosquito or fly vectors. PCR-based diagnosis of skin scrapings for *O. volvulus* (*224*) has also been shown to work, as has PCR of blood for brugian and bancroftian filariasis (*225*).

Diagnosis in the vector or intermediate host: Molecular xenomonitoring by PCR testing of blackfly or mosquito vectors has become an invaluable tool for epidemiological mapping of onchocerciasis (*201*) and filariasis, including in elimination programmes. However, as the intensity of infection decreases, the sample size of insect vectors that would be required to be analysed substantially increases (*226*). In practice however, the number of vectors that is recommended to be analysed in elimination programmes has been set at a constant level, with set thresholds being proposed in elimination settings.

Assessment of infection intensity: Aside from a semi-quantitative relationship between microfilarial load, as assessed by blood filtration or skin snip, and adult worm burden, there is a paucity of tools for quantifying intensity of infection. Palpation of onchocercal nodules (onchocercomata) as a tool for determination of infection prevalence and rapid epidemiological mapping of onchocerciasis (REMO) is only reliable in highly endemic areas. Community nodule prevalence has been used as a measure of community infection for onchocerciasis, by relating nodule to microfilarial prevalence. However, nodule palpation is relatively insensitive, particularly in areas of low endemicity (*227*), due to the fact that up to one half of *Onchocerca* nodules may be located in deep tissues rather than subcutaneously.

Response to antifilarial chemotherapy, including detection of anthelmintic resistance: Aside from assessment of microfilarial counts, diagnostics for establishing cure of filariasis are generally lacking, and as discussed above, the available drugs for MDA are not generally macrofilaricidal (with the exception of prolonged courses of doxycycline for long-term depletion of *Wolbachia* endobacteria (*132*)). This is particularly problematic when drugs with selective activity on the only life-cycle stage that is amenable to parasitological diagnosis – the mf – are used (e.g. DEC, IVM). Ultrasound in onchocerciasis may produce equivocal results (*228*). Thus, assessment of 'cure' after IVM therapy is problematic, and without other markers it hampers study of drug resistance. As IVM does not kill adult *O. volvulus* worms in the standard doses and dose intervals used in most control programmes, profiles of individual responses to IVM treatment have been studied by recording the rates of reappearance of mf in the skin at various time-points after administration of the drug, with faster than expected rates taken as indications of sub-optimal responses (*157*). As IVM treatment sterilizes adult female worms for a period after treatment, after several rounds of IVM (>4–6 rounds), the uterus of adult female worms should be free of motile mf three months after treatment. Embryograms of worms in nodules excised approximately three months after IVM treatment from subjects who have been treated repeatedly can be used as an adjunct measure of response to treatment (*157*). The problem of detection of anthelmintic resistance in filarial infections has been discussed in detail in section 4.2.3 above.

In LF, the detection of the 'filarial dance sign' in worm nests by ultrasound has been advocated to determine adult worm viability after macrofilaricidal chemotherapy (e.g. DEC, anti-*Wolbachia* therapy) (*229*). The disappearance of parasite antigen can also serve as a surrogate for cure (*222*).

Diagnostics for disease mapping and surveillance: Given the imperfections of current diagnostics for the filariases, particularly the invasive and insensitive nature of parasitological diagnosis and the often critical need to undertake cost-effective mapping, a number of novel techniques have been developed to overcome the shortcomings. For onchocerciasis, REMO began with work to identify proximity to blackfly vector breeding sites and community nodule prevalence (*198*). More recently, this has been supplemented by PCR screening of pools of flies (*201*), and the DEC patch test (*230*). For bancroftian filariasis, CFA assays in the form of immunochromatographic card tests (ICT) have been successfully incorporated into programmes to map its distribution (*223, 231*). The occurrence of SAEs following IVM distribution in areas where *L. loa* infection is highly prevalent (*232*) has required the development of model-based geostatistical methodologies (233–236) to map the risk of *L. loa* infection being above a predetermined prevalence (20%) in areas co-endemic for onchocerciasis.

Diagnostics in filarial elimination: The programmes to eliminate onchocerciasis from the Americas and LF on a more global basis have highlighted specific deficiencies in diagnostics for filariasis in elimination settings. Some relate to the problem of surveillance when infection prevalence falls to an extremely low level. Traditional parasitological methods are too insensitive, even if active case detection were logistically feasible. Xenodiagnosis by PCR has been deployed in this setting, both in PCR of flies in the Americas (*215, 237*) and of mosquitoes in Egypt (*53*), but may not be sufficiently sensitive at very low levels of transmission. Measuring the antibody response to specific recombinant proteins of these parasites has shown some utility in these settings (*215, 237*). However, such sero-epidemiological methods rely on the specificity of antibodies for the single or multiple parasite target antigens. In African settings where loiasis, bancroftian filariasis and onchocerciasis may all coexist, this problem may be of greater magnitude than in the Americas. While the results of these studies are encouraging, this approach poses significant logistical and financial challenges, and proof of success will only come after annual treatments have ceased and ongoing surveillance establishes that no new infections have occurred (*57*).

Diagnostics for mathematical modelling of filarial infection: A number of models including deterministic and stochastic approaches have been developed for onchocerciasis and LF. Work has also been conducted on investigating the dynamics of transmission breakpoints (*238, 239*). Some models of parasite genetic structure and drug susceptibility also exist for investigating the spread of anthelmintic resistance (*128, 240–243*), but the lack of molecular genetic markers of drug resistance and paucity of knowledge about its population genetics hamper further progress. Further research is crucial in this area, in particular molecular markers that can be used in models to aid prompt detection of heritable changes in drug efficacy, and preparedness to mitigate the effects of these on the ongoing control programmes.

The diagnostic landscape for filariasis is summarized in Table 5.

Table 5
Diagnostics for filariases

Objective	Lymphatic filariasis		Onchocerciasis	Loiasis
	Wuchereria bancrofti	*Brugia malayi*	*Onchocerca volvulus*	*Loa loa*
Parasitological diagnosis	Blood filtration for microfilariae (mf)		Skin snip	Blood filtration for mf
	Ultrasound		Nodule palpation	
			DEC patch test	
Antibody detection	✓	✓	✓	✓
Antigen detection	✓	N/A	N/A	N/A
PCR	Molecular xenomonitoring (PCR on mosquito [LF] or blackfly [onchocerciasis] vectors)			N/A
Assessment of infection intensity	Microfilaraemia intensity (e.g. mf/20µl)	Microfilaraemia intensity (e.g. mf/20µl)	Microfilaridermia intensity (mf/mg or mf/skin snip)	Microfilaraemia intensity (e.g. mf/ml)
	CFA level for adult worms		Nodule palpation for adult worms	
Assessment of drug efficacy	Disappearance of mf from blood (microfilaricidal efficacy) and rates of mf reappearance (anti-fecundity efficacy)	Disappearance of mf from blood	Disappearance of mf from skin (microfilaricidal efficacy) and rates of mf reappearance (anti-fecundity efficacy)	Disappearance of mf from blood
	Ultrasound changes in filarial nests	Ultrasound changes in filarial nests	Ultrasound changes in nodules	
	Clearance of CFA		Nodule histology	
Mapping	Antigenaemia prevalence		REMO	RAPLOA
Elimination	Seroepidemiology	Seroepidemiology	Seroepidemiology	N/A
	Molecular xenodiagnosis (mosquito PCR)		Molecular xenodiagnosis (blackfly PCR)	

✓ Available or method of choice; N/A, not available.
CFA, circulating filarial antigen; REMO, rapid epidemiological mapping of onchocerciasis; RAPLOA, rapid assessment procedure for loiasis; PCR, polymerase chain reaction; DEC, diethylcarbamazine.

4.4.2 Diagnostics for soil-transmitted helminthiases

Parasitological diagnosis: Infection with *A. lumbricoides*, hookworm (*N. americanus, A. duodenale*) and *T. trichiura* is diagnosed by detection of helminth eggs in stool using microscopic techniques. This is generally sufficiently sensitive, especially when a concentration step is included. Of note, it is not possible to differentiate between hookworm infection due to *A. duodenale* and *N. americanus* based on microscopic appearance of hookworm eggs. Kato-Katz thick smear allows the number of eggs per gram of faeces to be approximated. It is not, however, sufficiently quantitative to be reliable for assessment of anthelmintic efficacy (see below). In addition, the relationship between worm burden and egg output is not linearly proportional, with density-dependent fecundity resulting in the potential underestimation of adult worm burden, for example in *A. lumbricoides* infection (*244*).

Antibody tests: The use of antibody tests to detect parasite-specific antibody response, although possible, has not been considered necessary for diagnostic purposes.

Antigen detection: For antigen detection in hookworm infection some work has been undertaken in the zoonotic hookworm species *An. ceylanicum*, demonstrating the presence of coproantigen in the faeces (*245*). However, no assay has been reported for human hookworms.

Molecular diagnosis: PCR-based diagnosis of hookworm infection has been developed and has been subject to pilot testing in human populations (*246, 247*).

Intensity of infection: For STH, intensity of infection is a major determinant of morbidity, infection dynamics, and response to control, and would be best assessed by enumerating adult worm numbers. While this can be achieved by use of a cathartic in conjunction with an anthelmintic, preferably one that paralyses adult worms, such as pyrantel pamoate or levamisole, and enumerating parasites in collected faeces, this is not an easy test to perform routinely and is unreliable for hookworms and whipworms because of poor to moderate and variable efficacy of pyrantel and levamisole against these parasites (see Table 2, page 41). Therefore, most studies and surveys have relied on quantitative egg counting.

Of the quantitative methods described for egg counting, the Kato-Katz method is the most widely used and has undergone a number of validation studies (*248*). It has some methodological problems due to the fact that different helminth eggs, especially hookworm eggs, have different clearing times and viability. Hookworm eggs in particular are subject to lysis if the slides are not examined within 30 minutes. A preferred quantitative flotation technique in veterinary practice is the McMaster test (*249*). However, it is less well studied in human STH infections. Recently, a purpose-built flotation apparatus (FLOTAC®) has been designed and tested for the purpose of improving the quantitative analysis of faecal egg counts (*207*). Although FLOTAC® is more sensitive than the Kato-Katz technique (*250, 251*); it requires access to a basic centrifuge.

Response to anthelmintic chemotherapy including detection of anthelmintic resistance: The weaknesses in study design and consequent uncertainties in measures of STH anthelmintic drug efficacy have been recently reviewed (*138, 252*). These reports have highlighted the lack of standardization of diagnostic tests and measures of changes in infection intensity, as determined by reduction in faecal egg counts. While direct parasitological tests are relatively sensitive, their performance is sub-optimal at low intensity of infection, and therefore a single negative stool examination for helminth eggs may result in Type II errors in evaluation of trial outcomes. In veterinary practice, significant work has been undertaken to standardize assessment of anthelmintic drug efficacy (*253*), specifically in standardizing all aspects of the faecal egg count reduction test (FECRT). Assessment of drug efficacy by reporting reduction in egg counts is, in addition, subject to confounding due to the effect of density-dependent fecundity on egg counts (*254*). There may also be considerable geographic heterogeneity in the strength of density-dependent constraints on worm fecundity (*255*).

Pilot in vitro tests of anthelmintic response have been developed for hookworms where eggs passed in the faecal stream must mature into infective larvae before reinfection occurs (*143, 256*). While some work has been undertaken to standardize such tests (*257*), significant work remains. For *T. trichiura* and *A. lumbricoides*, it has not been possible to develop phenotypic tests due to the lack of egg hatch in the external environment, and an inability to readily assess parasite viability ex vivo.

Some work has been undertaken to develop molecular methods to genotype intestinal nematode parasites for genetic markers of anthelmintic resistance as discussed in section 4.2.3. Efforts have largely concentrated on genotyping for the specific polymorphisms in the β-tubulin gene, that are recognized to be associated with anthelmintic resistance in a range of veterinary nematodes, specifically mutations in the β-tubulin gene at codons 167, 198 and 200. Assay methodologies have been developed for *A. lumbricoides* (*134*), hookworms (*148, 149*) and *T. trichiura* (*134*) and the resistance-associated mutations have been found in some populations of these soil-transmitted nematodes. However, the relationship between the presence and frequency of these specific mutations and drug response phenotypes has not yet been fully characterized and is an important research priority so that fast and sensitive genotyping analyses applied to pooled egg samples can serve as surveillance tools for anthelmintic resistance.

Disease mapping and surveillance: As infection with these parasites is less subject to geographic variations in prevalence, and qualitative diagnosis is relatively easy, no specific problems in infection mapping are present.

Diagnostics for mathematical modelling: A number of mathematical models based mainly on differential equations for adult worm burden have been developed for the population dynamics and control of intestinal nematodes (*258*). Given current difficulties in accurately quantifying worm burden, such models may not account sufficiently for this uncertainty, a consideration that is seldom recognized. The relationship between infection and morbidity has also been studied in some models, with the assumption that the latter is linearly proportional to the former (*259*). Most of these models have been developed to mimic endemic equilibrium situations, and then used to simulate the effects of control interventions (*260*). Further work as described below is required to fit models to intervention data and to understand the effect of immunological memory on infection.

The diagnostic landscape for STHs is summarized in Table 6.

Table 6
Diagnostics for soil-transmitted helminths

Objective	A. lumbricoides	N. americanus An. duodenale	T. trichiura	S. stercoralis
Parasitological diagnosis	Stool microscopy with or without concentration step[a]			+/-
Coproculture	Harada Mori for specific identification of hookworms			Coproculture
Antibody detection	N/A	N/A	N/A	✓
PCR and antigen detection	Experimental			
Assessment of infection intensity	Quantitative faecal egg count, PCR (experimental)			N/A
Assessment of drug efficacy	Clearance of eggs from stool. Commonly used indices are the cure or clearance rate (CR; the proportion of people who become egg negative after treatment), and the egg reduction rate (ERR; measured by the faecal egg count reduction test [FECRT; the proportional reduction in egg count after treatment in comparison to that just prior to treatment])			Negative coproculture Decline in antibody titre

[a] By sedimentation (e.g. formalin-ethyl acetate sedimentation or flotation (e.g. ZnSO4)).
✓ Available or method of choice; N/A, not available; +/-, acceptable but not ideal.

4.4.3 Diagnostics for schistosomiasis (including infections by *Schistosoma mansoni*, *S. haematobium* and *S. japonicum*)

Parasitological diagnosis: Parasitological diagnosis of *S. haematobium* infection is readily undertaken by urine filtration. While urine is easily collected, due to the circadian pattern of egg excretion, specimens should ideally be collected between 10:00 am and 2:00 pm, and preferably after physical exercise. Diagnosis of intestinal schistosomiasis (*S. mansoni* and *S. japonicum*) is generally made by examination of stool specimens. The Kato-Katz thick smear method is the standard method recommended by the WHO for both qualitative and quantitative diagnosis of intestinal schistosomiasis. Its main advantage is that it is a highly specific, relatively simple and inexpensive (estimates in Uganda put the cost as ~USD 2.00 per test), even under field conditions. However, it requires trained technicians and specialized equipment such as microscopes. Furthermore, it produces semi-quantitative egg counts that can be used as surrogates of infection intensity. However, like many other parasitological tests, if only a single Kato-Katz slide is prepared from a single stool specimen, sensitivity is reduced particularly in light infections. This leads to a marked underestimation of the prevalence of *S. mansoni* infection especially in areas where prevalence is low, and likewise can confound confirmation of cure after chemotherapy (*261, 262*). To overcome the lack of sensitivity of the parasitological methods (urine filtration and Kato-Katz technique) in situations of low worm burden, replicate urine or stool samples, or a number of Kato-Katz slides prepared from a single (or sequential) stool sample, are required. However, this increases costs, may hamper survey logistics due to the need for repeated collection of stool samples, and would complicate control strategies based on mass screen and treat (MSAT) strategies.

For *S. haematobium* infection, the presence of micro- or macrohaematuria has enabled the development and validation of a range of indirect diagnostic tests useful for epidemiological mapping of prevalence, such as the dipstick methods which detect micro- and macro-haematuria. Simple interview methods to ascertain a history of haematuria have also been shown to be useful. For example, the WHO-supported Red Urine Study as well as others have established the utility of a simple oral questionnaire for history of haematuria, to estimate the prevalence of infection among school-age children (*263, 264*).

Antibody tests: Patent schistosome infection is highly immunogenic and anti-schistosome antibodies can be readily detected by a wide array of techniques. Currently, the ELISA technique using soluble egg antigen (SEA) as the target is the most widely used technique (*265–267*). Other techniques are also used (*209*). However, serodiagnosis of schistosomiasis suffers from a number of drawbacks common to antibody detection techniques for parasite infection (*265*): a) it does not accurately reflect the presence of active infection, with parasite-specific antibodies remaining for a long time after cure; b) it does not reflect infection intensity; and c) it has poor specificity (i.e. a high proportion of egg-negative, antibody-positive results).

Nevertheless, immunodiagnostic techniques represent the best available methods for diagnosis in areas of low intensity of infection where the sensitivity and specificity of these methods appear to be satisfactory.

Antigen detection: Schistosome antigens are present in serum and urine of infected subjects (*268*). According to their migratory behaviour in immunoelectrophoresis, they are commonly referred to as circulating anodic antigens (CAA) and circulating cathodic antigens (CCA). These two circulating adult worm antigens are the basis of antigen capture immunoassays (*269*). Measurement of CAA in the blood, serum, and urine by ELISA-based assays is both sensitive and specific, and is subject to significantly less interassay variability than egg counts (*270*). The CCA assay has been further developed as a of point of care urine ELISA dipstick (*271*). In field evaluation studies, the test was unexpectedly insensitive for detection of *S. haematobium* infections (*272*), but performed relatively well for *S. mansoni* infection (*272*). There was a correlation between intensity of *S. mansoni* infection, as measured by egg counts and CCA concentration (*272*).

Molecular diagnosis: The application of PCR as a technique for the detection of schistosomiasis has been explored for *S. mansoni* and *S. japonicum* in human faeces and urine (*210, 273*). The technique has been evaluated as a diagnostic tool for schistosomiasis in areas of medium and low intensity of infection. While PCR-based assays are very sensitive and specific, like parasitological techniques they can also be subject to sampling errors in stool specimens.

Snail intermediate host: The geographic distribution of schistosomiasis is directly related to the distribution of the appropriate susceptible snail intermediate hosts for the corresponding schistosome species. *Biomphalaria* susceptibility to *S. mansoni* infection varies according to the different snail age classes, genetic variation, immune system status and geographic areas where both snails and trematodes occur (*274*). Molecular-based methodologies have been proposed to be used to support snail morphological analysis. These techniques can also be used for evaluation of molluscs, specifically for detection of infection, including pre-patent infection, differentiation of human pathogens (*S. mansoni* and *S. haematobium*) from other trematodes, and detection of infection in dead snails (*275*).

Intensity of infection: Estimation of the intensity of schistosomiasis infection is an essential requirement but one for which available diagnostics are insufficient. Intensity of schistosomiasis is an important indicator for: a) monitoring and evaluation of control programmes; b) assessment of efficacy of anti-bilharzial drugs; and c) as the most important determinant of morbidity.

Urine filtration technique is the standard technique for estimation of intensity of *S. haematobium* infection, while the Kato-Katz technique is the standard method for quantitative diagnosis of intestinal schistosomiasis. However, due in part to the overdispersed nature of schistosome egg output in stool, and daily variation in excretion, as noted above it has been recommended that replicate faecal/urine samples be collected over several (ideally a minimum of three) consecutive days to quantify infection intensity. This is especially the case in low endemicity settings, in monitoring of control programmes, and in chemotherapy efficacy trials (*261, 262*). However, such approaches are not logistically or financially feasible except in research settings. Statistical methods have been proposed to improve accuracy in the parasitological estimates (*261*).

Response to anthelmintic chemotherapy including detection of PZQ resistance: At present, the main objective of schistosomiasis control is to reduce or eliminate morbidity, or at least serious disease. MDA of PZQ is the main tool for morbidity control strategy. Unfortunately, a number of reports from endemic areas have suggested, although not confirmed, that resistance or tolerance to PZQ might exist in *S. mansoni* in Egypt (*276*) and Senegal (*277, 278*), thus highlighting the need for sensitive diagnostic techniques for monitoring and evaluation of control programmes and for monitoring the efficacy of PZQ chemotherapy. Presently, monitoring the efficacy of PZQ in schistosomiasis relies on the relatively insensitive method of measuring reduction in egg excretion following treatment (*279*). In addition to any variations in drug effect on the worms, several factors can confound the interpretation of such studies. These include variability in pharmacokinetics of PZQ in different individuals, the confounding effect of variability of the host immune responses to the worms, and the maturity of worms (PZQ is relatively ineffective against juvenile worms) (*277, 280*). While a number of approaches to overcoming the significant impediments to detecting drug resistance using clinical efficacy as the parameter have been reported, none can be readily deployed at programmatic levels. These have included transfer of clinical isolates from human patients into mice for testing (*281, 282*), and the development of in vitro tests for PZQ sensitivity of schistosomes (*283–285*), and miracidia (*283*). While adoptive transfer into mice has enabled detailed laboratory study, it is not always successful, is expensive and requires sophisticated infrastructure.

Disease mapping and surveillance: As the epidemiology of schistosomiasis is characterized by focal variation in distribution, with large-scale patterns of transmission that are influenced by climatic and local environmental conditions, the integrated use of geographic information systems (GIS), remote sensing and geostatistics has provided important insights into its ecology and epidemiology on a variety of spatial scales (*7*). Nevertheless, the microecology of snail and parasite endemicity may be difficult to define without detailed parasitological surveys (*286*).

Elimination: To date, most schistosomiasis control programmes in SSA have been aimed at morbidity reduction rather than elimination of infection. As the prevalence of schistosomiasis decreases, the need for improved diagnostic approaches for surveillance purposes will inevitably increase. In the PRC, where programmes aim at elimination of *S. japonicum*, high sensitivity serologic tests (indirect haemaglutination assay (IHA), ELISA, or dipstick) are used to screen for evidence of likely infection; positive cases are followed by parasitologic stool examination (using Kato-Katz). Notwithstanding the results of the parasitologic tests, all seropositive cases receive empiric PZQ therapy.

Diagnostics for mathematical modelling of infection: Mathematical modelling of schistosomiasis is a field that has attracted a great deal of attention, and a large number of models exist that are based on prevalence of infection (*107, 287*), intensity of infection (*288*), deterministic (e.g. EpiSchisto (*289*)) or stochastic (e.g. SCHISTOSIM (*290*)) approaches. Variability in egg output has received considerable attention (*291*), as well as its relationship with infection prevalence and intensity (*292*). A positive and statistically significant relationship between serum concentration of CCA and CAA (as measures of worm burden) and egg output has been reported (*293*); such relationships have been used to confirm density-dependent fecundity in *S. mansoni* (*294*). More recently, attention has focused on modelling studies of the impact of chemotherapy on parasite genetic diversity and drug resistance (*295–297*).

The diagnostic landscape for schistosomiasis is summarized in Table 7.

4.4.4 Diagnostics for taeniasis (*Taenia solium*/cysticercosis)

Parasitological diagnosis: Microscopic diagnosis, by identification of *Taenia* eggs in stools, even with use of concentration methods, is relatively insensitive. Moreover, as the eggs of *T. solium* and *T. saginata* are morphologically identical, the identification of *Taenia* eggs in stool samples should be reported as *Taenia* spp. eggs. In general, copro-parasitological diagnosis of taeniasis is not recommended unless there is a specific indication and no suitable alternative is available. While it is theoretically possible to distinguish proglottids of *T. saginata* from *T. solium* by counting the number of uterine branches, this is not an easy test to perform.

Antibody tests: Stage-specific antibody-detecting immunoblot techniques have been developed for adult tapeworm infection (*298*). These are reported to have very high sensitivity and specificity, with the caveat of an unknown duration of seropositivity after cure or parasite death. Immunoblot using purified glycoprotein antigens is the assay of choice for serological diagnosis of cysticercosis, with very high sensitivity and specificity. This test, however, relies on parasitic cysts as a source of antigens, and thus assays using recombinant or synthetic antigens are currently under development (*299*).

Antigen detection: Coproantigen detection ELISA greatly improves the diagnostic sensitivity of taeniasis (*300*). Unfortunately, the availability of this assay beyond research settings is very limited. Monoclonal antibody-based ELISA assays to detect circulating parasite antigen are available for diagnosis of cysticercosis. Such assays confirm the presence of live parasites. However, such tests seem to be only moderately sensitive in individuals with only one or two brain cysts.

Molecular diagnosis: Stool PCR can differentiate *T. solium* from *T. saginata*. There is a paucity of information about the sensitivity of PCR-based assays for diagnostic purposes (*301*).

Intermediate host: Porcine cysticercosis serves as a marker of endemicity, with pigs representing an important reservoir of taeniasis.

Intensity of infection: Most (>90%) human tapeworm carriers harbour a single tapeworm, and human infection with more than two tapeworms is extremely rare (*302*). In porcine cysticercosis and apparently also in human cysticercosis, most infected individuals carry a few parasites and individuals with heavy infection are uncommon. It is not known whether persistence of taeniasis in populations is mostly driven by the majority of pigs, that are infected with few cysts (and thus difficult to detect), or by the few pigs with many cysts (potential source of infection to many people if eaten).

Response to anthelmintic chemotherapy: The efficacy of chemotherapy for tapeworm infection is generally assessed by parasitologic examination of stool, which has the drawbacks noted above. Assessment of cure of neurocysticercosis generally requires serial neuroimaging studies.

Mapping and disease surveillance: Surveillance is best focused on assessment of porcine cysticercosis for two reasons: a) it is much more prevalent than human infection; and b) it changes more rapidly due to the much faster replacement of the pig population compared to the human population.

Elimination: While proof of concept of the feasibility of actively eliminating transmission has been recently obtained in Northern Coastal Peru, tools for diagnosis in an elimination setting are required, that are less costly, simple, and exportable to other settings (*303*).

The diagnostic landscape for schistosomiasis and taeniasis is summarized in Table 7.

Table 7
Diagnostics for schistosomiasis and taeniasis

Objective	Schistosomiasis			Taeniasis
	Schistosoma mansoni	*Schistosoma haematobium*	*Schistosoma japonicum*	*Taenia solium/ T. saginata*
parasitological diagnosis	Stool Kato-Katz	Urine filtration	Stool Kato-Katz	Stool microscopy with or without concentration
Antibody detection	✓	✓	✓	+/-

continues

Table 7 continued

Objective	Schistosomiasis			Taeniasis
	Schistosoma mansoni	Schistosoma haematobium	Schistosoma japonicum	Taenia solium/ T. saginata
Antigen detection	+	+/-	N/A	+/-
PCR	Experimental			
Assessment of infection intensity	Stool Kato-Katz (eggs per gram of faeces [epg])	Urinary egg count (eggs per 20 ml of urine)	Stool Kato-Katz (eggs per gram of faeces [epg])	N/A
Assessment of drug efficacy	Clearance of eggs from stool	Clearance of eggs from urine	Clearance of eggs from stool	N/A
Mapping/ elimination	Seroepidemiology	Seroepidemiology	Seroepidemiology	N/A

✓ Available or method of choice; N/A, not available; +/-, acceptable but not ideal.

4.5 Issues related to bringing new diagnostics to market

As outlined in the section above there is a significant literature on prototype diagnostic tests for helminth infections. Once a prototype diagnostic device for a "neglected tropical disease" such as a helminth infection reaches an acceptable level of technical performance, its further development beyond proof-of-concept requires that a range of significant challenges be overcome.

Foremost, there is the likely limited interest in commercialization, a consequence of the restricted financial return, due to the low priority for specific diagnosis of most of these conditions in endemic settings; secondly there is the low royalty for licensing (304); and thirdly, there are the significant costs associated with the commercial scale manufacture and marketing of such tests. Furthermore, the expectation that diagnostic tests gain regulatory approval from the US Food and Drug Administration (FDA) (305) or the European Union Medical Device Safety Service (MDSS) (306) likely requires significant investment. A minimum requirement for purchase is evidence of good manufacturing practices as documented by either compliance with ISO 13485:2003 or 21 CFR 820 from the FDA. While gaining formal regulatory approval may not be essential for the deployment of a new diagnostic test for helminth infections or other NTDs, such approval carries significant advantages as it is likely to be easier to gain support from donors and funders for an approved diagnostic test that can be used in the context of a public health control programme.

Despite these challenges, examples exist of diagnostic devices or platforms relevant to helminth infections that have successfully reached market. These include CFA tests for filariasis (*220, 221*), and the urinary CCA for schistosomiasis (*271*). Not well documented in the scientific literature are the difficulties each of these platforms experienced in reaching market and maintaining a presence.

Examination of the landscape of diagnostic tests and their pathway to deployment indicates that the standard commercial pathway is not well suited to the needs for diagnostics to aid in the control of helminth parasites. A novel approach that can be used possibly as a model is the one created for the diagnosis of tuberculosis, sleeping sickness, and malaria: the Foundation for Innovative New Diagnostics (FIND) (*307*), an example of Product Development and Implementation Partnership (PDIP). Recently, PATH, an international nonprofit organization that improves the health of people around the world, and the University of Washington established The Center to Advance Point-of-Care Diagnostics for Global Health, which has as its goal to advance the development of diagnostic tests for patients in low-resource settings around the world. Funded by the National Institute of Biomedical Imaging and Bioengineering of the National Institutes of Health, the Center will support development of technologies through clinical testing, identification of innovative technologies, assessment of critical clinical needs, and a training programme.

As is outlined by Tony Murdoch in the online monograph "A Diagnostic Path to a Better World" (*308*), a range of complex issues need to be dealt with to successfully develop such diagnostics. The analysis identified the following issues: 1) identifying specific patients' needs in developing countries and targeting products to all levels of the health system; 2) understanding the market – the potential volumes, distribution of products and end-users' profiles; 3) arranging the financial considerations to ensure they cover both research and development costs; 4) settling issues regarding intellectual property rights for products with no or limited financial return; 5) finding the right manufacturing approach and harnessing possibilities for technology transfer; 6) creating methods for evaluating the product through clinical trials and for introducing it at country level; 7) working with governments to adapt national policies and approaches; 8) working with local laboratories to ensure they have the capacity to use the products effectively; and 9) working with donors and national governments to make sure tests can be purchased at prices affordable to all. These approaches will be essential for the successful development of the novel diagnostic tests needed for the control of helminth parasites. However, even if such a model for development of diagnostic tests were implemented, a system would need to be put in place to finance procurement. Requiring the end-user to pay for such diagnostic tests would likely result in the tests not being used.

4.6 Advances in mathematical modelling of helminth infections

Mathematical models have an important role to play in our understanding of the processes underlying observed helminth epidemiological patterns. They have been useful for providing insight into the mechanisms (such as the operation of parasite density dependence) responsible for infection persistence, resilience and stability. Very few models, however, have been used to seriously inform helminth research or policy and decision-making in the context of control programmes. An exception to this is possibly the use of the simulation model ONCHOSIM by the OCP (*309*). Fewer models, if any, have been used to investigate or prepare for emerging/re-emerging infections, public health research and control challenges. This paucity is limiting our ability to understand and predict the behaviour, under anthropogenic or natural change (including control interventions and climate change), of multi-host parasite systems, multi-parasitized host populations, and parasites with complex transmission routes; transmission involving various vectors or intermediate hosts; and the spread of strains resistant to interventions including insecticides, molluscicides, anthelmintic drugs or vaccines.

Population dynamic models seek to describe the changes with respect to time (and host age where appropriate) of parasite abundance (infection prevalence and intensity) and derived measures (presence of active infection, parasite exposure, morbidity) in humans and intermediate hosts or vectors at baseline (endemic equilibrium) and during an intervention. They are based on our current understanding of the parasites' population biology and transmission dynamics, and describe how the life-stages in the definitive host, environment (for STHs), or intermediate hosts/vectors (for schistosomiasis and the filariases) are inter-connected in the parasite's life-cycle through contact, transmission, establishment and parasite fecundity rate. Models can be deterministic or stochastic, population-based or individual-based, and may track infection intensity and/or prevalence (*310, 311*).

Most of the helminth models that have been developed pertain to single parasitic infections in closed populations, and very few have been fitted to data obtained through monitoring and evaluation (M&E) of large-scale control programmes including MDA. The majority ignore the possible development of resistance to the selection pressures imposed by the interventions on populations of parasites, vectors, and intermediate hosts.

With increasing use of advanced statistical methods (including Bayesian approaches) that can be implemented given the current availability of faster and more potent computing power, parasite epidemiology researchers are fitting dynamic models to data for estimation of unknown parameters of interest. In particular, this has permitted estimation, given the data, of parasite life-span (*312, 313*), treatment efficacy and drug effects on different parasite life-stages (*97, 314, 315*), variation in host immune response to parasite life-stages (*316*), and transmission parameters, which otherwise are elusive to direct observation/ experimentation. Recent examples are in the field of multi-host models for schistosomiasis japonica (measuring the transmission from hosts to snails and from snails to hosts) (*107*); schistosomiasis mansoni (measuring the reductions in force of infection as a result of implementation of the SCI in Uganda) (*59*); identification of sub-optimal responses to IVM in onchocerciasis (*127*).

Epidemiological and risk mapping integrates observed, georeferenced data and predictive, remote-sensing derived, environmental variables into (Bayesian) geostatistical modelling to indicate areas with different probabilities of infection presence and severity across chosen geographical scales, aiding national control programmes to evaluate the extent of the public health problem posed by helminth infection and deploy appropriate anthelmintic strategies (*70, 122, 317–321*).

Recently, mathematical models of parasite population dynamics have been modified to incorporate parasite genetic structure with regard to drug susceptibility in filarial infections (*128, 240, 242, 243*). These models have permitted theoretical exploration of the spread of putative resistance alleles in filarial populations under various assumptions of the genetics of drug resistance and parasite inbreeding. Such frameworks constitute a good example of how mathematical models can aid programme preparedness, as they are now ready to be modified and developed in the directions required for control and elimination of these infections. As part of the M&E strategies, models can also help in the design of treatment efficacy and effectiveness studies, as in the characterization of sub-optimal responses to IVM (*127*) and identification of molecular genetic markers for the study of parasite genetic structure and prompt detection of reduced anthelmintic efficacy (*128*). With regard to schistosomes, a model including time delays, parasite mating structure, multiple resistant strains, and complexity in the parasite's life-cycle has been used to explore the impact of drug treatment on survival of resistant strains (*295, 297*). In other models, resistance has a cost in terms of reduced reproduction and transmission. The likelihood that resistant strains will increase in frequency depends on the interplay between their relative fitness, the cost of resistance, and the degree of selection pressure exerted by drug treatments (*296, 297*).

4.7 Advances in the understanding of pathology and assessment of morbidity

Filariasis: An important advancement in the study of pathogenesis by filarial nematodes is the discovery of the parasites' endosymbiotic *Wolbachia* bacteria, which play an important role in the causation of inflammatory-mediated filarial disease. The development of acute and severe inflammatory responses in people infected with *B. malayi* and *O. volvulus* is associated with the release of *Wolbachia* into the blood following death or damage of the worms after anti-filarial chemotherapy (*322, 323*). Lymphoedema (LE), the severe pathology of filariasis, affects only a minority of the 120 million people infected with LF. The majority of infected individuals develop filarial-specific immunosuppression that starts even before birth in cases where mothers are infected and is characterized by regulatory T-cell responses and high levels of IgG4, thus tolerating high parasite loads and microfilaraemia (*324*). In contrast, individuals with this pathology show stronger immune reactions biased towards Th1, Th2 and probably also Th17. Importantly, innate immune responses that are triggered by filarial antigens, and specifically *Wolbachia* endosymbionts, ultimately result in the activation of vascular endothelial growth factors (VEGF), thus promoting lymph vessel hyperplasia as a first step to LE development. Hydrocoele, a pathology with some similarity to LE in which both lymph vessel dilation and lymph extravasation are shared sequelae, has been found to be strongly associated with a VEGF-A SNP known for upregulation of this (lymph) angiogenesis factor (*324*).

Onchocercal skin disease (OSD): The accepted clinical classification and grading system of Murdoch et al. (*325*) defines and describes the various cutaneous changes and resulting lesions associated with *O. volvulus* infection, namely, acute papular onchodermatitis (APOD), chronic papular onchodermatitis (CPOD), lichenified onchodermatitis (LOD), skin atrophy (ATR), depigmentation (DPM, also known as leopard skin), troublesome itching (pruritus), and lymphatic involvement (LYM) plus hanging groin (HG). The scheme has now facilitated a variety of large-scale prevalence surveys, drug trials, psychosocial and economic studies, and selection of clinical groups of patients for detailed immunological and genetic studies (*15*).

Onchocerciasis and epilepsy: A recent study investigated the association between onchocerciasis and increased risk of epilepsy and found that epilepsy prevalence increased, on average, by 0.4% for each 10% increase in onchocerciasis prevalence. These results provide further evidence that onchocerciasis is associated with epilepsy, and suggest that the disease burden of onchocerciasis might have to be re-estimated taking into account this relationship (*326*).

Onchocerciasis, blindness and excess human mortality: The relationships between microfilarial load and blindness incidence, and microfilarial load and excess human mortality, have been investigated in the area covered during 1975 and 2002 by the OCP in West Africa (*13*). A recent analysis concluded that the excess relative risk of mortality is density dependent and more elevated in children (*327*).

Soil-transmitted helminths: The three main STHs, ascariasis, trichuriasis, and hookworm, can cause common clinical disorders in humans. The gastrointestinal tract of a child living in poverty in a less developed country is likely to be parasitized with at least one, and in many cases all three STHs, with resultant impairments in physical, intellectual, and cognitive development. In STH infections, the occurrence of disease is directly related to the intensity of infection and is highest in school-age children. However, in the case of hookworm infections, high intensity is generally reached in adulthood, aggravating iron-deficiency anaemia in women of reproductive age. High intensity of infection is associated with high morbidity and the risk of severe complications, such as intestinal obstruction. In childhood, hookworm contributes to moderate and severe anaemia in school-aged children, and there is increasing recognition of a similar contribution in preschool children. Cross-sectional evidence from Africa and Asia shows that 30%–54% of moderate to severe anaemia in pregnant women is attributable to hookworm, and intervention studies suggest that antenatal anthelmintics substantially increase maternal haemoglobin concentrations as well as birthweight and infant survival (*66, 328*). Focus should now be on developing regular periodic chemotherapy programmes for children and women to control morbidity, and its use should be optimized to sustain drug efficacy; targeted treatment of high-risk groups, treatment at frequencies appropriate to the nematode generation time, and use of combinations of anthelmintic drugs are all strategies to reduce and delay selection of resistant strains.

STHs do not elicit protective host immunity at first infection, establishing chronic infections during the host's life, and, in the case of hookworm, intensity of infection rises with the age of the host. STHs are thought to survive within the host not just by warding off immune attack, but also by aggressively subverting the host immune response to create niches that optimize successful residence, feeding and reproduction. The survival of STHs suggests that they succeed by achieving some form of balanced parasitism, in which transmission is maintained and acute morbidity avoided. This ideal homeostatic state almost certainly needs an environment rich in regulatory mechanisms, some of which are now being more clearly understood. Much of the survival success of STHs can be attributed to their secretomes, which interact with host tissues and maintain the parasitic existence, specifically the secretions that modulate the host's immune response. For example, an adult *N. americanus*-derived protein that binds selectively to natural-killer cells is able to induce these cells to secrete interferon-γ in the gut, which would potentially counteract the development of a potentially host-protective Th2 response that might eliminate the parasite. Other immunomodulators have also been described. Other hookworm pathogenesis-related proteins combat haemostasis by binding to platelets and inhibiting their activation. The molecules that *Ancylostoma* secretes to inhibit host coagulation and ensure blood flow and continuous bleeding at the site of parasite attachment, including novel inhibitors of factor Xa and VIIa/tissue factor, have also been described in detail, as has a multienzyme cascade involved in host red-blood-cell lysis and haemoglobin digestion. *Ascaris* secretes from its body wall a pepsin inhibitor that is thought to protect maturing worms from digestive enzymes in the stomach before they reach the small intestine. *T. trichiura* secretes large amounts of a protein called TT47 that forms ion-conducting pores in lipid bilayers, allowing the parasite to invade the host gut and maintain its anterior end in a syncytial environment in the caecal epithelium (*66*). The characteristics and subsequent development of the acute primary inflammatory and immune responses in very young humans to STH infection is now an important component of research studies and should provide a better understanding of their pathogenesis and identify possible targets for vaccines and/or other control measures.

Schistosomiasis and other trematode infections: The most severe pathology associated with these infections is cancer. The association between *S. haematobium* and bladder cancer is strong and consistent. The eggs of *S. haematobium* provoke granulomatous inflammation, ulceration, and pseudopolyposis of the bladder and ureteral walls. Chronic lesions can then evolve into fibrosis, and carcinoma of the bladder (squamous cell carcinoma).

There is currently no agreement regarding the measures that should be included in schistosome morbidity assessment (*329*). However, several techniques have been used for estimation of *S. haematobium* morbidity: 1) urinary egg counts; 2) haematuria; 3) albuminuria; and 4) measurement of eosinophil cationic protein (ECP). Webster and colleagues, in a discussion of morbidity markers that were evaluated within all SCI activities across selected SSA countries (*31*), reported that measurements of parasitological intensity, combined with haemoglobin/anaemia counts and ultrasonography, performed best as schistosomiasis-related morbidity indicators. In addition, the urinary albumin excretion profile was a promising measure that was considered worthy of ongoing research (*67*). Additional measures that were evaluated but considered less reliable included distended stomach, umbilical circumference, anthropometric measurements and health questionnaires.

Pathogenesis of liver fluke-associated cholangiocarcinogenesis involves chronic inflammation and oxidative DNA damage (*115, 330*). The liver fluke endemic area of Khon Kaen, Northeast Thailand, has reported the highest incidence of the liver cancer in the world (*331*). Three helminth parasites – *Opisthorchis viverrini, Chlonorchis sinensis, S. haematobium* – have been designated as Group 1 carcinogens (metazoan parasites that are carcinogenic to humans) by the International Agency for Research on Cancer, WHO (*332, 333*). Therefore, not only do these trematodes cause pathogenic helminth infections, but they are also carcinogenic in humans in a similar fashion to several other more well-known biological carcinogens, in particular hepatitis viruses, human papilloma virus and *Helicobacter pylori*.

4.8 Analysis of the challenges for epidemiological data and mathematical models

4.8.1 Transmission thresholds

The basic reproduction ratio (R_0) represents the threshold condition for parasite invasion and persistence; it has to be greater than 1 for the parasite population to reach its endemic state. For the vector-borne filariases it is possible to calculate threshold biting rates below which the infection would not persist and which, in part, depend on the proportion of bites that are taken on humans (*334–337*), emphasizing the role of measures to reduce vector density and vector-human contact. However, by definition R_0 is a somewhat idealized, parasite density-independent entity. In reality, many transmission processes do depend on parasite density, with the effective reproduction ratio (R_E) reflecting the changes in transmission potential of a parasite with parasite density (*238, 338*). For dioecious parasites (separate sexes) and in those host-parasite systems with facilitating types of density dependence there will be unstable equilibrium parasite densities (transmission breakpoints), below which the parasite population would, in principle, become locally extinct (because females will not be mated and/or parasites will not establish), and above which the parasite population would return to endemic equilibrium. The value of R_E will be equal to 1 both at endemic equilibrium (each female worm in the population replaces itself) and at the unstable transmission-breakpoint equilibrium. Understanding the behaviour of the host-parasite system in the vicinity of the breakpoints is an area of important research that requires the concourse of mathematical analysis and knowledge of vector-host-parasite interactions and parasite epidemiology. The values of both threshold biting rates and parasite breakpoints are themselves complex dynamic entities dependent on the nature and magnitude of vector- and host-specific density-dependent processes, the local characteristics of vector competence and vectorial capacity in different vector species, and the degree of parasite overdispersion among hosts in the population (*238, 239, 338, 339*). This highlights the problems faced in trying to obtain a single, one-size-fits-all threshold transmission or infection breakpoint value that can be applied across the board, and suggests that the end-game in parasite elimination programmes will have to be flexible and adapt to the locale-specific microepidemiology of infection in endemic communities (*239*).

4.8.2 Parasite population biology factors

Epidemiologically, helminth infections of humans are characterized by persistent, insidious, long-lasting and often polyparasitic infection, frequently exhibiting high prevalence in the affected populations (*258*). This is due to the long life-spans of the parasites (e.g. *O. volvulus*, *W. bancrofti*, *Schistosoma* spp., other trematodes, cestodes); to repeated and to some extent cumulative infection

(*O. volvulus*, lymphatic filariae, trematodes, cestodes); and to rapid reinfection (*Schistosoma* spp., *A. lumbricoides*, *T. trichiura*, hookworm) (*258, 340*). Many regions are endemic for more than one parasitic helminth species due to commonalities in biology, ecology, transmission routes, and environmental and behavioural determinants of transmission (*286, 341*). Yet knowledge is scarce as to whether these associations between different species generate or are caused by biological interactions (among helminth species and between helminth and other infections) within individual hosts, and how they contribute to shaping epidemiological patterns of infection and morbidity (*342–345*).

Human helminthiases are highly stable and resilient. In contrast to other infections, e.g. viral diseases that are characterized by marked epidemic population cycles, time-limited interventions that may lead to dramatic reductions in prevalence of the parasite infection are quickly followed by re-emergence and eventual restoration of the parasite population to baseline levels (*346, 347*).

Of particular importance is the pattern that emerges when population infection prevalence is plotted against infection intensity for a wide range of examined populations and helminth infections. The prevalence vs. intensity relationship is usually strongly non-linear, initially increasing rapidly and soon reaching a high prevalence associated with a wide range of infection intensities, particularly in areas of intense transmission (*336, 348, 349*). The wide range of prevalence-intensity values reflects a high degree of spatial heterogeneity in the distribution and abundance of helminth infections at various levels of geographical scale, and the importance of understanding both the macro- and microepidemiology of these infections for effective deployment of locale-specific interventions (*317, 318, 350–352*).

The distribution of parasite burden is highly heterogeneous among host populations, with a relatively small fraction harbouring heavy infection, and most harbouring light and moderate infection. The consequences of such distribution include: 1) the contribution to disease burden and transmission potential of different groups in the population can be highly heterogeneous; 2) such distribution and any post-intervention variation influence the stability of the host-parasite relationship and the regulation of parasite population abundance, with the most heavily infected hosts contributing the most to such regulation (*258, 353*); 3) infection may persist in populations for prolonged periods driven by small sub-groups of hosts who harbour enough parasites to keep the life-cycle going and who would need to be identified, targeted and monitored with anthelmintic treatment (*63, 258, 353*). This is a particularly important issue in the elimination phase of control programmes. As more is learnt about the genomics of parasites, a greater appreciation is being gained of the heterogeneity within parasite species, which may contribute to heterogeneity of infection between hosts, to variation in response to treatment and ultimately to the potential for drug resistance to develop.

The implications of this include: 1) control programmes need to monitor both the prevalence (presence) and intensity (quantity) of infection present in areas under control; 2) infection prevalence may decrease more slowly than intensity, particularly in the initial phases of control; 3) the shape of the prevalence vs. intensity relationship may change during control (because of changes in underlying parasite distributional patterns) (*354, 355*). This can represent a considerable challenge to control programmes, particularly as they advance; infection load and incidence decrease, and diagnostic methods lose their ability to detect active infection as discussed in more detail in section 4.4.

4.8.3 Co-infections, multiple populations, and niche-shifts

Although many of the populations afflicted by helminthiases are poly-parasitized or co-infected with other pathogen species, most models consider the dynamics of single-species parasite populations. Most models also ignore explicit spatial structure and are confined to closed populations of hosts, parasites, and vectors. More recently however, models for investigation of the population dynamic consequences of co-infections (*356–359*), of multiple, spatially heterogeneous populations (*360*), and of connected (meta-) populations (*361*) are starting to receive attention. These frameworks constitute important scientific advances for our understanding of: the effects of interventions affecting some parasite/vector species or zoonotic reservoirs more strongly than others; the efficacy of integrated NTD control; and the ability of some parasites, pathogens, intermediate hosts or vectors to invade/occupy niches previously used by those species which are most vulnerable to particular interventions.

4.8.4 Infection and disease mapping

Research efforts should be undertaken to determine optimal strategies for rapidly and simultaneously assessing a number of NTDs to implement integrated control approaches. In addition to mapping single infections, efforts should also be devoted to develop risk mapping and prediction of co-infections to aid integrated and cost-effective control (*70, 287, 321*). However, although useful for initial assessment of distribution and endemicity level of the infections prior to the implementation of control, rapid epidemiological assessment (REA) and mapping methods may not offer enough flexibility to reflect parasite population changes effected by the interventions (e.g. nodule prevalence in onchocerciasis, the mainstay of REMO, may not adequately reflect changes in the viability and contribution to transmission of adult worms during a control programme).

4.8.5 Morbidity control vs. elimination

Although the goal of some programmes has been that of morbidity control and elimination of the public health burden imposed by the diseases (STHs, schistosomiasis and onchocerciasis in Africa), others aim at interruption of transmission and eventual elimination of the parasite reservoir (LF, onchocerciasis through vector control/elimination in Africa, onchocerciasis in Latin America). The models to inform parasite elimination should generally be stochastic because, as parasite density decreases, stochastic variations (and stochastic fade-out) will be more important than the mean behaviour. It will be important to investigate the influence of factors such as initial endemicity level and transmission intensity; host heterogeneities (exposure/susceptibility/predisposition) and resulting parasite overdispersion; vector/intermediate host competence and vectorial capacity (including vector density, efficiency, and biting rate); treatment frequency, duration and coverage required; synergistic effects of vector/snail control, etc.

Whereas morbidity control may benefit from age-targeted chemotherapy (of those hosts at higher risk of acquiring heavy infection), parasite elimination will require prolonged mass treatment of all those infected at all endemicity levels (and in all endemic communities if parasite eradication is aimed at). This strategy will substantially shrink the size of susceptible parasite refugia (populations of untreated parasites, not subjected to chemotherapeutic pressure) (362), increasing the chances of anthelmintic resistance. Parasite elimination programmes that rely on chemotherapy must therefore put in place careful surveillance systems for prompt detection of transmission resurgence and monitoring of drug susceptibility. The same applies for those programmes relying on vector/snail control because of the possibility of insecticide/molluscicide resistance.

4.8.6 Transition from endemic to post-control parasite biology and ecology

Most of our parasite population biology understanding and modelling efforts have focused on the study of endemic situations (288, 335, 363–367). Those frameworks that explore the impact of control scenarios do so based on the same assumptions made when describing the behaviour of the host-parasite systems at endemic equilibrium, and for genetically homogeneous populations (259, 368–376). Very few models, and these only recently, are being fitted to data systematically collected during the interventions (when initiatives have had the foresight to follow up substantial cohorts of individuals through time) (59), or incorporate genetic variability (upon which the selection pressures imposed by control will surely act) (128). This may be explicable given that the impetus for global parasite control and elimination efforts has truly gained momentum in the 21st century. Entering the second decade of the 21st century, and despite global financial difficulties, it is hoped to move into a period of sustained parasite control and elimination where possible. However, it must be stressed that the mainstay of the current programmes is based on chemotherapy with a very limited arsenal of affordable or donated drugs, vulnerable to the development of resistance, and mostly unknown with regard to their modes of action and long-term impact on human helminth infections.

Apart from a few exceptions (*377–380*), there is a striking paucity of models for the transmission dynamics, control, and morbidity due to cestode infections, which needs to be urgently addressed also in light of climate change and its impact on agricultural and farming practices.

It is necessary to revise assumptions about the processes that regulate reinfection, investigate the long-term impact of changes in exposure and parasite acquisition/mortality on host immune responses, explore the prolonged effects of anthelmintics on the biology, particularly the parasite reproductive biology and mating structure (*295*), and improve our understanding of the relationship between infection and disease, to better inform those programmes that aim at morbidity control.

For those programmes that aim at elimination, models should seek to reflect the decreased sensitivity of the measures currently used for infection assessment, aid the epidemiological interpretation of complementary serological (antibody and antigen) measures, quantify the contribution to transmission of ultra-low parasite densities, and inform surveillance sampling protocols. Also, the synergistic effects of adjuvant chemical and non-chemical means of parasite control (including vector and snail control, vaccination, mop-up strategies, environmental modification and health education) should be explored and exploited. Mathematical models have a greater potential than has been realized to date to provide evidence-based decision-making tools to support anthelmintic control programmes. A greater disposition for dialogue and mutual understanding is needed between the architects of such programmes, their implementers in endemic countries, and the mathematical and population biologists developing the models. A continuous dialogue between quantitative epidemiologists and those implementing control programmes, and recognition that modellers and statisticians should be involved from the outset during the early phases of funding applications, programme design and implementation, and subsequent M&E, would iron out many difficulties and help realize the potential of models to become fully embedded into parasite control strategies.

4.9 Advances in helminth biology

4.9.1 Parasite genomics and functional genomics

The recent research landscape for helminth parasites has been dominated by rapid progress in genome sequencing of several nematode and trematode parasites of significance to human disease. Today, the genome sequences of 22 species of helminths that either infect humans or are closely related parasites are completed or under way including most or all of the significant STHs, schistosomes and filarial species (*381*). A comprehensive genome analysis has been published for several of them, including the lymphatic filarial nematode *B. malayi* (74), the dog hookworm *Ancylostoma caninum* (382), and the blood flukes *S. japonicum* and *S. mansoni* (90, 383). Indeed, the cost of sequencing using 2nd generation technologies is such that obtaining a genome sequence is no longer expensive, and it should no longer be seen as a major barrier or significant investment. Importantly, the genome of *O. volvulus* is now being sequenced by the Sanger Center. However, as discussed above, the available genomes are either poorly annotated, or not annotated at all, and there are almost no tools available with which gene function can be tested directly. For example, the current genome drafts of *S. mansoni* and *S. japonicum* achieve five- to six-fold coverage of the entire genome; however, this includes large numbers of incontinuous contigs and supercontigs with gaps (77). This immediately raises difficulties with identifying the transcriptome of these trematodes and also identifying genetic polymorphisms shared between closely related species (384).

The tools used to test gene function are broadly defined as "functional genomics" tools, i.e. tools with which gene function can be investigated. The relatively primitive state of tool availability for helminths contrasts markedly with, for example, the situation with several groups of protozoan parasites (especially *Plasmodium* spp.) where the development of functional genomics tools has accompanied genome sequencing. This has resulted in much more useful annotation of protozoan parasite genomes, and the genomes have yielded information that has been applied to practical ends (e.g. the creation of a comprehensive database that contains a list of all potential drug targets for malaria (385)). Databases such as this have led to the establishment of the UNICEF/UNDP/World Bank/WHO Special Programme for Research and Training in Tropical Diseases (TDR) Drug Target Prioritization Network which has developed an open source database of drug targets (386) covering multiple disease pathogens in support of target selection for rational drug design (387). This database is now providing the engine for establishing an in silico screening network as well as an innovative high throughput screening approach for infectious tropical diseases.

Provided that similar, effective functional genomics tools are developed for helminths, available genomics data will have a major impact in the long term. This report seeks to define some of the tools it may be useful to develop, the areas in which the impact of applying these tools might be felt, and the research steps that are required to achieve that impact. It will also discuss other aspects of helminth biology where, in our opinion, basic research is needed if new treatments are to be developed and current treatments made more effective and sustainable.

Functional genomics tools fall into two broad categories: 1) bioinformatics tools for sequence mining to generate hypotheses concerning likely biological function, and 2) experimental tools with which gene expression can be manipulated in the target organism (or, in the case of parasites, also the host) and with which the consequences of this manipulation for the biology of the parasite and its relationship with the host can be observed and measured.

The first bioinformatics tools that are applied are generally genome-wide homology searches, usually using variants of BLAST to generate automatic annotations based on sequence homology. While perhaps useful as a tool with which to assess genome content, homology-generated gene annotations are at best a very rough guide and at worst downright misleading. Furthermore, in parasites the limited utility of a homology-based approach is undermined further by the poor performance of gene-finding software in parasite genomic sequence. Nonetheless, several relatively sophisticated bioinformatics tools with which, for example, functional classes can be grouped or putative metabolic pathways predicted, have been published recently along with examples of their application. These could be used to, for example, search for likely differences between the parasite and its host that may offer the opportunity for either vaccine or drug development, or to search for molecules which may mediate host pathology (*381*). Allied to these bioinformatics tools is the dramatic increase in sequencing capacity, with deep "whole transcriptome" sequencing yielding quantitative as well as qualitative data on parasite gene expression. These data will aid in gene finding and annotation as well as point to key regulatory events in the parasites' relationships with their hosts.

The development of tools with which parasite gene expression can be directly investigated has also been the subject of recent developments. RNA interference (RNAi), whereby gene expression is knocked down, has been described for several parasitic nematode and trematode species, but only for a single monogenean and a single cestode. The effectiveness of RNAi in helminths seems to be extremely variable, and it remains to be seen whether it is a generally useful technique, or whether its application will be restricted to a handful of susceptible species (*381*). The alternative means by which gene function can be decreased is via loss of function mutation. The converse of knock-down of expression is manipulation of expression by gene knock-in. There are now a number of reports of either transient or heritable transgenesis in several species of parasitic nematodes and trematodes (three of which are parasites of humans) (*381*) and in at least one cestode (*388*). The recent advances in transgenesis, especially in *Echinococcus multilocularis*, offer some hope of reverse genetic analysis via gene knockout. Other techniques that have been developed for a few of the helminths are whole-mount in situ hybridization and microarray analyses, but their use is limited for the functional analysis of helminth-encoded genes (*389, 390*).

Advances in helminth genomics have also shed light on a wide range of helminth-derived immunomodulatory proteins that regulate host processes. The expression of these proteins varies depending on the life phase of the helminth, making effector profiles difficult to trace, especially in instances of polyparasitism. Also, some of these proteins have components that have high sequence identity with their mammalian orthologs, indicating that helminths may exploit some human proteins for their own benefit. For instance the genomes of *B. malayi* and *Schistosoma* spp. reveal the presence of predicted components of Ras-Rad-MAPK and TGF-B-SMAD signaling pathways including fibroblast and epidermal growth factors, suggesting the possible exploitation of host factors for their own growth and development (*77, 383*). Detailed studies in comparative genome analysis are hence also required to identify helminth-dependent gene products that are responsible for the majority of the observed pathology in both human and animal disease.

One of the goals of genome-scale analyses is to elucidate the basic biology of helminths, including of host-parasite relationships, that is relevant to human disease. Broadly, this biology can be divided into transmission biology, immunology, and host-parasite interaction/pathology, as detailed below.

4.9.2 Transmission biology

Recent advances in transmission biology relate largely to the development of complex models for parasite population dynamics and the beginnings of investigation of the population genetics of a few species (section 4.8). The few population genetics studies of helminths suggest that, not surprisingly, the nature of the parasite's life-cycle has a very significant impact on the population genetics, often with perhaps unexpected results. Furthermore, the population genetics of a given species may be different under different circumstances (e.g. *S. mansoni* populations in different epidemiological settings show different genetic structures). Modelling suggests that differences in population structures will affect transmission and, among others, the selection and spread of drug resistance alleles.

4.9.3 Immunology

Parasites and hosts interact primarily via the host immune system. Work over the past several years in parasite immunology has focused to a large extent on the identification of mechanisms of protective immunity and vaccine development, but the emerging theme in basic research is the realization that the host-parasite immunological relationship is interactive, and that helminths are masterful immunoregulators. Immune regulation by parasites includes suppression, diversion, and alteration of the host immune response, resulting in an anti-inflammatory environment, which is most favourable to parasite survival. A characteristic feature of helminth infection is a Th2-dominated immune response, but stimulation of immunoregulatory cell populations, such as regulatory T cells and alternatively activated macrophages, is equally common. Typically,

Th1/17 immunity is blocked and productive effector responses are muted, allowing survival of the parasite in a "modified Th2" environment. Successful immunoregulation also limits collateral damage to the host. The remarkable range of parasite life histories, transmission strategies, and physiological niches is reflected in the variety of immunomodulatory activities targeting key receptors or pathways in the mammalian immune system observed across the three taxonomic categories (nematodes, cestodes, and trematodes) of helminths (391). The mechanisms that initiate and sustain this immune regulation remain incompletely understood, but are clearly important to consider because mass chemotherapy programmes alter the dynamics of transmission and the burdens of infection in affected communities and also have the potential to reverse these immunoregulatory effects. Such a change could also have unintended consequences for global elimination efforts, such as increased susceptibility to infection or to patency, increased disease burden in children, or increased morbidity caused by the targeted helminth and concurrent infections.

Furthermore, increasing attention is being paid to studying poly-pathogen infections in which infectious agents interact in a synergistic or inhibitory fashion, thus having a significant impact on pathogenesis or the maintenance of health of those who are co-infected. For example, it has been proposed that individuals infected with parasitic helminths have increased susceptibility to malaria infection (43, 392), and that helminth infections may alter susceptibility to clinical malaria (393, 394). There is now increasing interest in investigating the consequences of co-infection (42) and assessing whether mass deworming affects the incidence of clinical malaria. This is however not a new research topic. Nearly thirty years ago it was suggested that infection with the intestinal nematode *A. lumbricoides* was associated with the suppression of malaria symptoms and that anthelmintic treatment led to a recrudescence of malaria (395, 396).

Concurrent helminth infections have also been shown to alter optimal vaccine-induced responses in the human host; however, the consequences of this condition have not been adequately studied especially in the context of a challenge infection following vaccination. Demands for new and effective vaccines to control chronic diseases like tuberculosis, HIV, and malaria as well as deploying vaccines for the so-called childhood diseases in Africa require a systematic evaluation of confounding factors that may limit vaccine efficacy, such as the presence of co-infections with helminths in populations of humans targeted for vaccination. The bias towards a Th2 cytokine milieu induced by helminth infection, especially the notable depressing of interferon (INF)γ, has been compared to an "anti-adjuvant", which is pivotal in cellular immune responses (393, 397). It has been shown that the presence of helminths may alter the host's response to by-stander antigens like the tetanus toxin vaccines (398–400) probably due to polarization of the immune response to a Th2-like response or the production of immunomodulating cytokines like interleukin (IL)10 that dampen both Th1 and Th2 responses. The *A. lumbricoides* reduced response to the oral cholera vaccine could be, however, restored by ABZ treatment (*401*). The potential impact of helminth infections on trials of novel vaccines such as tuberculosis and malaria will have to be considered (*402, 403*).

Most importantly, it must be remembered that most of the anthelmintics currently being used are not totally curative, and numerous rounds of MDA may be necessary to reduce the levels of infection below those necessary to sustain transmission. It can therefore be anticipated that such major alterations in the levels of infection in endemic communities might have a dramatic impact on the degree of their immunity to the targeted parasites and other co-infections, resulting in either a higher degree of protection against re-infection (thereby promoting success of the MDA), or conversely, resulting in less protection (and becoming a potential impediment to elimination). For example, studies in humans and cattle have shown that *Onchocerca* infected hosts in which infections were cleared by chemotherapy acquired new infections of equal or higher intensity than those exhibited before the therapeutic intervention (*404–406*). Therefore, for example, in areas where MDA with IVM does not result in transmission interruption, those who are re-infected might develop higher burdens of infection. Better understanding of the host-parasite immune relationships at play at the molecular level and at different life-cycle stages within the host is thus important not only to make more precise predictions about the eventual success of the specific elimination efforts, but also to alert the MDA programmes to potential problems that might arise from altered immunity in treated communities.

4.9.4 Host-parasite interaction and pathology

Although approximately one billion of the world's population is plagued by helminthiases, very little is understood in terms of host-parasite interactions. Helminths have evolved to co-adapt and evade host defense mechanisms and it is these intricate interactions that have made them such successful pathogens. The disease becomes overt only when the worm burden (or intensity of infection) exceeds a certain (but mostly unknown) threshold; it is the factors controlling this delicate balance in the interaction between helminths and their hosts (intermediate and definitive) that still require extensive research. Helminth factors and host responses that induce pathologies are key determinants for disease manifestations. Investigations on helminth biology at molecular (genetics, transcriptomics, proteomics) and cellular levels as well as host immune/inflammatory responses therefore are important for understanding disease pathogenesis (*381, 407, 408*). This will undoubtedly improve clinical management and lead to novel strategies for both diagnosis and treatment. Therefore, helminth biology research is fundamental for informing and underpinning prevention and control of helminth infections.

Since most helminthiases result in chronic infection, severity of pathology depends on the number/types of parasites, host immune responses/genetics and duration of infection. Acute infection infrequently occurs among endemic populations but is common among visitors or migrants and after primary infections. For some parasites, as the infection moves from the initial acute phase to a chronic phase, inflammatory responses may resolve, leaving many patients asymptomatic, but in a proportion of patients (which varies in different host-parasite relationships) the acute initial phase is followed by chronic inflammation. These chronic inflammatory responses often do little or no damage to the parasites, and in the case of penetration of the eggs of *S. mansoni* through the intestinal wall, are actually exploited by the parasite to its advantage. Modulation of host immune responses by the parasites is a likely explanation for many of these phenomena, but the details of the transition from acute to asymptomatic versus chronic inflammation are generally unknown. Helminths, their eggs and excretion-secretion products can directly induce host pathology in many infections. Liver flukes (*Fasciola hepatica*, *Opisthorchis* spp. and *Clonorchis sinensis*) use their suckers (oral and ventral) to hook onto bile-duct epithelium for nutrition and migration (*409–411*), causing ulceration. *Fasciola* proteases can degrade host tissue, forming abscesses during the migration phase (*409*).

Proteomics analysis of proteins secreted by infective larvae, immature flukes, and adult *F. hepatica* has shown that proteolytic enzymes, cathepsin L, cathepsin B, and asparaginyl endopeptidase cysteine proteases as well as novel trypsin-like serine proteases and carboxypeptidases, which cause pathology, are developmentally regulated. Proteases such as FhCL3 and cathepsin B have specific functions in larvae activation and intestinal wall penetration, whereas FhCL1, FhCL2, and FhCL5 are required for liver penetration and tissue and blood feeding (*412*). Excretion-secretion products from the human liver flukes *Op. viverrini* and *C. sinensis* can induce cell proliferation in vitro (*413, 414*). Similarly, live filarial parasites or filarial antigens induced significant human lymphatic endothelial cell (LEC) proliferation. Moreover, serum from patently infected (microfilaria-positive) patients and those with longstanding chronic lymphatic obstruction induced significantly increased LEC proliferation compared to sera from uninfected individuals (*415*). Live, intact *S. mansoni* eggs secrete a soluble factor that stimulates human umbilical vein endothelial cell proliferation (HUVE) in vitro in a manner similar to crude soluble egg antigen (*416*). Overall, most helminth proteins have mitogenic effects on a variety of cells and may directly induce cell proliferation, providing insight into the mechanisms underlying the pathology seen in helminthiases such as lymphangiogenesis (LF), neovascularization (schistosomiasis), or biliary proliferation (opisthorchiasis and clonorchiasis).

O. volvulus and the lymphatic filariae habour intracellular *Wolbachia* bacteria, now recognized as an obligatory symbiont essential for reproduction and survival of the worm, and therefore emerging as a novel target for chemotherapy. Both parasite and endobacteria contribute to onchocerciasis and LF pathogenesis and morbidity. Both genomes and excretory-secretory (ES) proteomes of *B. malayi* and its *Wolbachia* are known (*74, 93, 417*). Molecules have been identified that promote inflammatory or counter-inflammatory immune mechanisms, divert the host's immune response, or promote parasite evasion (*91*). Future studies will help to understand *Wolbachia*'s role in pathogenesis. Differences in *Wolbachia* abundance between the savannah and forest forms of *O. volvulus* may help explain differences in ocular pathogenicity (*418*).

4.9.5 Vector-filaria and snail-schistosome interactions

Of all the helminthiases in this report, the filarial nematode and the trematode infections are the ones with complex life-cycles involving a vector or a snail host, respectively. This interface is not of trivial importance given the close biological association that exists between the parasites and their invertebrate hosts. Yet, vector/intermediate host-parasite interactions are usually under-appreciated though they may hold the key to many of the evolutionary and epidemiological underpinnings of these infections.

For the filariases, the issues involved are ingestion of the skin- or blood-dwelling mf, their survival and development into infective L3 larvae (there is no multiplication of the parasite within the vector), and, in common with all vector-borne diseases, survival of the vector until completion of the extrinsic incubation period and beyond. These processes have been investigated from genetic, immunological, physiological, and ecological perspectives in an effort to understand the basis for susceptibility/refractoriness to the parasites by the corresponding arthropod taxa (e.g. mosquitoes in LF, blackflies in onchocerciasis), and the close association between vector biting behaviour and the availability of microfilariae (mf) to be ingested from blood or skin. From a population biology point of view, some of these underlying processes translate into relationships between consecutive parasite life stages that are of interest for epidemiological models. Some of these relationships (e.g. the number of *O. volvulus* or *W. bancrofti* L3 larvae per fly or per mosquito as a function of the microfilarial load on which the insects were fed) may be nonlinear, indicating the operation of density dependence. As described in section 4.6, density-dependent processes regulate parasite population abundance and their effect is relaxed as a result of anthelmintic treatment, leading to enhanced per parasite probabilities of transmission. Therefore, an understanding of vector-parasite interactions becomes even more crucial as control programmes progress from morbidity reduction to elimination goals. Also, in some settings, there may be various vector-parasite combinations whose features may be impacted differently by interventions (e.g. different effects of antivectorial measures depending on whether the vector species feed and rest indoors or outdoors, or have a propensity to feed on humans or non-human hosts). See Griffin et al. (*419*) for a theoretical exploration in malaria, but similar issues will arise and need research in LF, particularly where both infections are transmitted by the same *Anopheles* vectors.

Microfilariae of lymphatic filariae show differential periodicity in the peripheral circulation of the definitive host, according to host endogenous circadian factors and also to whether mosquito biting is nocturnal (e.g. nocturnally periodic *W. bancrofti* transmitted by *Culex* or *Anopheles* spp.) or diurnal/vespertine (e.g. diurnally periodic or sub-periodic *W. bancrofti* transmitted by *Aedes*, and in the Andaman and Nicobar islands of India by *Ochlerotatus niveus* mosquitoes) (*420*). For a review of vector-parasite interactions in onchocerciasis and their epidemiological and evolutionary implications, see Basáñez et al. (*238*). Bockarie et al. (*421*) discuss a variety of vector issues and vector-parasite relationships relevant to LF transmission and elimination.

Unlike the filariases, schistosome transmission occurs via free-swimming larval stages, cercariae, infective to mammalian definitive hosts, and miracidia, infective to the molluscan intermediate hosts. These non-feeding larvae obtain their energy through limited glycogen reserves, so there are strong selective pressures to locate and penetrate a suitable host rapidly post-emergence. Some of the snail-parasite issues in the schistosome life-cycle are similar to those of the filariases, highlighting the importance of parasite survival and development to the infective stage, and the survival of the intermediate host. In addition, schistosome larvae must themselves locate their subsequent hosts and asexually reproduce within the snail. Schistosome miracidia have evolved effective snail-seeking behaviours (*422, 423*), e.g. *S. mansoni* miracidia show geonegative and photopositive responses whereas *S. haematobium* show geopositive and photonegative responses, directing them, respectively, towards their contrasting *Biomphalaria glabrata* and *Bulinus globosus* snail host habitats.

Young/recently hatched miracidia of ~1–3 hours exhibit dispersal strategies rather than host attraction (*424*), potentially limiting density-dependent constraints occurring in the snail hosts. Density trade-offs appear to occur throughout the parasite's life-cycle (*425*). Miracidia have also been demonstrated to show sympatric specificity for host location (*426*) and penetration (*427*).

Once successful penetration of a suitable snail host has occurred, schistosomes undergo migration, asexual reproduction and emergence of cercariae whilst evading the snail's immune response. Trade-offs often occur between daily cercarial production and host longevity, life-history traits and virulence, with lower daily shedding associated with higher host survival and longer infectivity (*425*). Intra- and inter-specific interactions also affect life-history responses, with *S. mansoni* mixed strain infections inducing greater snail mortality in comparison to single strain infections (*428*).

Cercarial emergence can vary in its chronobiological rhythm to maximize the chances of encountering a suitable definitive host. These interactions are also affected by inter-specific and intra-specific variation (*429*). Lu et al. (*430*) have shown that in *S. japonicum*, which can infect up to 40 definitive host species, cercarial emergence from rodent infections peak at dusk and dawn, when their hosts are most active, whilst cercarial emergence for bovine strains peaks at noon.

Schistosome snail hosts are hermaphroditic, so even with intense mollusciciding or drought, they can still repopulate from extremely low numbers. However, the host-specificity shown by the Egyptian strains may have contributed to explaining why mollusciciding alongside mass PZQ treatment was successful, with no long-term resistance emerging within Egypt (*431*). Thus, an understanding of snail-schistosome interactions may be crucial for identifying optimal control mechanisms.

4.10 Analysis of challenges stemming from gaps in knowledge of basic helminth biology

Current global efforts to control or eliminate helminth infections, focusing principally on the reduction of transmission using MDA, may reduce infection rates in the short to medium term, but may also have undesirable effects on the evolution of host immune responses and thus on disease presentation. For example, reductions in levels of endemicity following MDA might lead to diminished immunoregulation and consequent exaggeration of disease immunopathology after re-infection. Repeated treatment itself might trigger exaggerated host immune responses to parasite products (e.g. the Mazotti reaction in onchocerciasis) that could enhance progression of disease and result in persistent damage or even cancer development. Even with a decrease in overall prevalence of infection, persistent, low-level infections could result in altered immunoregulatory and/or inflammatory responses that could, in turn, affect an individual's susceptibility to other types of infection, or reduce responsiveness to vaccines. Several SAEs may occur after drug treatment of onchocerciasis and LF (discussed above). PZQ treatment of the human liver fluke *Op. viverrini* induces severe acute inflammatory response and oxidative DNA damage of the bile duct epithelium due to parasite burst (*432*). Repeated infections with the liver fluke induce more severe DNA damage (*433*). This suggests that repeated treatments and infections may induce intermittent severe inflammation and DNA damage leading to carcinogenesis in endemic areas subject to MDA.

4.10.1 Host-parasite interaction and immunopathology

Host responses to helminth parasites are important factors in disease manifestation. Typically, pathological characteristics may manifest initially as acute reactions that may be followed by chronic inflammation that results in significant immunopathology, much of the disease being due to the host's response to the presence of the parasite rather than the direct action of the parasite. Primary infection in naïve hosts often results in acute disease manifestation. For some parasites, as the infection moves from the initial acute phase to a chronic phase, inflammatory responses may resolve, leaving many patients relatively asymptomatic or suffering from subtle morbidity, but in a proportion of patients (which varies in different host-parasite relationships) the acute initial phase is followed by chronic inflammation. These chronic inflammatory responses often do little or no damage to the parasites, and in the case of penetration of the eggs of *S. mansoni* through the intestinal wall, are actually exploited by the parasite to its advantage. Modulation of host immune responses by the parasites is a likely explanation for many of these phenomena, but the details of the transition from acute to asymptomatic versus chronic inflammation are generally unknown.

Onchocerciasis and lymphatic filariae: In onchocerciasis the interaction between *O. volvulus* and the host's defence system is vital to the individual's tolerance of the infection. Different immune responses to *O. volvulus* cause considerable variation in the clinical manifestations of human onchocerciasis. Onchocercal lesions result from inflammatory reactions involving immunological mechanisms; the role of the immune system in the pathology is demonstrated by the accelerated worm destruction (mf stages) that occurs during microfilaricidal chemotherapy. Microfilarial destruction can be mediated by antibodies to the surface-associated antigens of the worm and enhanced by complement. Recently, the role of *Wolbachia*, an endosymbiont essential for filarial worm fertility and survival, has been implicated in the immune response to and pathogenesis of filarial infections (*91, 322, 323, 434, 435*), and inflammatory responses following treatment of filariae with DEC or IVM have been suggested to result in part from the release of high numbers of endobacteria from degenerating tissue mf (*405, 436*). *Wolbachia* and their products are reported to elicit pronounced innate immune responses in vitro and this is known to be mediated by monocytes/macrophages and neutrophilic granulocytes (*437–439*). Brattig et al. (*440*) have shown that a *Wolbachia*-derived distinct protein (WSP) can elicit in vitro inflammatory responses consistent with those observed previously in treated filariasis patients.

Adverse reactions following microfilaricidal therapy have been associated with potent innate responses including release of TNF-α and IL-6, as well as the presence of *Wolbachia* DNA in the blood, liberated from mf after treatment. The levels of inflammatory cytokines are shown to correlate with the presence and amount of *Wolbachia* DNA (*441, 442*). In a mouse model, *Wolbachia* constituents have been implicated in inflammatory reactions leading to corneal opacity and stromal thickening (keratitis), with the involvement of toll-like receptor (TLR)4 signalling (*443*). *Wolbachia*-associated molecules have been shown to participate in the interaction between the filarial parasite and the human host. WSP, using

TLR2 and TLR4 for immune cell stimulation, might activate both the innate and the adaptive immune system of the host. Thus, filarial nematodes, through their endobacteria, acquire characteristics of bacteria and signal immune responses via TLR. Th1-type inflammatory responses in filariasis may therefore depend on the endobacteria dormant in the parasite (*440*).

On the other hand, immunoepidemiological data provide evidence that humans can acquire protective immunity against *O. volvulus* infection (*195, 444–447*); this appears to be directed against molecules of invading L3 larvae. In onchocerciasis hyperendemic areas, some individuals remain without detectable signs of disease despite heavy exposure to transmitting vectors for years, and this type of immunity is directed against developing infective larvae. These individuals have been termed 'putatively immune' (PI), and a strong cellular reactivity of their peripheral blood mononuclear cells (PBMC) to *O. volvulus* extract in vitro suggests pre-exposure to *O. volvulus* antigens (*446*). A better understanding of how MDA with IVM will affect pathology and immunity is needed.

Schistosomiasis: Exacerbation of host pathology occurs in some infected individuals and this may be explained by host genetics/immunogenetics. In chronic schistosomiasis, severe hepatosplenic pathology occurs in less than 10% of the infected population. The pathology is characterized by excessive deposition of collagen and other extracellular matrix components around schistosome egg granulomas in the liver, causing periportal fibrosis and progressive occlusion of the portal veins (*448*). In murine schistosomiasis, the pathology is induced by a CD4+ Th2 driven granulomatous response directed against schistosome eggs lodged in the host liver. The Th2 cytokines IL-4 and IL-13 drive this response, whereas IL-10, IL-13Rα2, IFN-γ and a subset of regulatory T-cells act to limit schistosome-induced pathology. A variety of cell types including hepatic stellate cells, alternatively activated macrophages and regulatory T-cells have also been implicated in the pathogenesis. Current knowledge suggests the immunopathogenic mechanisms underlying human schistosomiasis are likely to be similar (*449*). Moreover, host genetic background also plays a pivotal role in determining the susceptibility to and outcome of schistosome infections (*450–452*). For example, segregation analysis of a Brazilian population has revealed that susceptibility to infection is controlled by the 'SM1' ('*S. mansoni* 1') gene locus that has been linked to the 5q31–q33 chromosome region comprising the genes for IL-4, IL-5 and IL-13 (*453, 454*). Another study involving a Sudanese population indicated that the segregation of a co-dominant gene (SM2) could account for the familial distribution of severe *S. mansoni* schistosomiasis in this population. Linkage analysis indicated that this gene occurred within the 6q22–q23 region with polymorphisms close to and in the IFN-γreceptor 1 gene (IFNGR1) (*452*). A better understanding of factors that influence infection, pathology (including anaemia due to chronic inflammation) and protection is needed.

Other trematode infections: In other trematodiases, severe fibrosis of affected tissues/organs is also a hallmark of chronic infection in certain individuals. Advanced periductal fibrosis around the intra-hepatic bile ducts in *Op. viverrini* infected people is associated with elevated parasite-specific IL-6 production among 11 Th1/Th2 cytokines, in comparison to those with no or minimal fibrosis (*455*). Moreover, the fibrosis occurs in a small subset of infected populations. Detailed studies on molecular pathogenetic mechanisms of the liver fluke trematodes need to be conducted.

The few studies on detailed pathogenesis of trematode infections including their associated cancer have shown, for example, that prevalence of cholangiocarcinoma antigens differs among different geographical regions even within the same country. The diversity of parasite genetics/intermediate hosts should be explored in correlation with cancer incidence if there are any carcinogenic strains of the parasites. Morbidity in infected individuals is also different and only a small proportion of infected individuals develop cancer. Host genetics/immunogenetics is a key factor of susceptibility. Detailed studies on the pathogenesis/immunopathogenesis and host-parasite interaction among individuals with different genetic background are of priority for research. A better understanding of the pathogenetic mechanisms will lead to primary and secondary prevention of the diseases.

Cestode infections: For cestodes, cysticercosis caused by *T. solium* larvae is a major public health problem, especially in the developing world, and NCC is considered to be the most common parasitic infestation of the central nervous system (*456, 457*). Approximately 25% to 50% of active epilepsy cases in the developing world including India and Latin America are due to NCC (*458*). NCC induces neurological syndromes that vary from asymptomatic infection to sudden death. Neuroimaging is the mainstay of diagnosis. The genome project of *T. solium* has been started (*459*) and knowledge of the genetic structure of *T. solium* is being applied to epidemiology, transmission and pathogenicity of this disease (*460*).

Studies on innate and acquired immune responses in human *T. solium* NCC over decades have highlighted conditions that appear to be favourable for the survival or destruction of the parasite and for the benefit or injury to its host (*461*). In addition, animal immunological models of cysticercosis – *T. crassiceps* in mice, and *T. solium* in pigs – add more information on immune regulation of cysticercosis. The parasite is able to manipulate the host immune system into supporting its survival by keeping a low inflammatory profile caused by the production of some cysticerci-released products that have immunomodulatory activities. Moreover, the mouse model has been used to design vaccine strategies, some of them with promising results (*462*). Further aspects of research are the role of the host's immune response in: 1) developing an acute inflammatory response around the parasite, which is strongly associated with symptoms, and seems to mark the onset of the process of parasite death; 2) developing perilesion oedema in old, calcified lesions (this is also strongly correlated with new symptomatic episodes); 3) controlling and eliminating infection, most likely in mild exposed individuals; and 4) mechanisms allowing the parasite to modulate the immune system at the central nervous system level and survive for years.

4.10.2 Other aspects of basic biology

Basic biology research should inform and underpin the prevention and treatment of helminth infection. The possible list of basic research issues is very long indeed, but there are four broad areas that stand out as central to the development of the next generation of helminth control measures. Advances and challenges stemming from research gaps in the following areas have been discussed above in section 4.9.

Functional genomics: The recent research landscape for helminth parasites has been dominated by rapid progress in genome sequencing of several nematode and trematode parasites of significance to human disease. Perhaps most notable amongst the now sequenced species are the trematodes *S. mansoni* and *S. japonicum*, while amongst the nematodes, genome sequences are either available, in progress, or planned for >15 species of human health importance, including most or all of the significant STHs and filarial species. Although the cost of sequencing is no longer prohibitive, the annotation of available genomes is poorer than desirable for the development of useful tools with which to directly test gene function, as discussed earlier in this report. Without annotation and functional genomics tools, the sequence data are not truly useful, so careful thought should be given to investing not only in sequence generation but also in annotation. The underdeveloped state of functional genomics tools for helminths is in sharp contrast with the situation for protozoan parasites, and *Plasmodium* spp. particularly. As pointed out above, genome sequencing, accompanied by the annotation of protozoan parasite genomes and the subsequent development of functional genomics tools, has enabled the generation of testable gene function hypotheses. The results of such experimental tests of function are now being applied to practical ends such as parasite genetics investigation, and drug and vaccine development. A similar, genome-driven expansion of schistosome research is gathering momentum as a result of developments that have followed the publication of annotated schistosome genomes and concurrent development of better tools with which those genome sequences can be utilized. Research funding for translational basic research will follow the development of tools with which fundamental questions can not only be posed, but also answered. What is required is "seed" funding to develop the genomics resources. The available genomics data could have a major impact in the long term provided that similar, effective functional genomics tools are developed for other helminths (especially for nematodes). Without functional genomics tools, the potential impact of the sequence data will be much diminished. Therefore, renewed energy and resources need to be devoted not only to generating helminth sequence resources but also to annotating those sequences, especially to developing tools with which the function of helminth genes can be tested experimentally, and to supporting work on other aspects of helminth biology such as transmission and infection, immunology and pathology.

Transmission biology: The major challenge here is that despite the acknowledged importance of parasite population biology and population genetics for understanding parasite transmission, relevant data are sparse for most helminth species. This is especially problematic when attempting to monitor the impact of control measures such as MDA on parasite populations, their structure and reproductive biology, the incidence of new infections and how this may be affected by the relaxation of any density-dependent processes that may operate (including acquired immunity), and the potential for the selection and spread of resistant genotypes. Once again, the experience from malaria, where drug resistance selection and spread is recognized and accepted as an inevitable consequence of drug administration, suggests that the development of tools with which to monitor the selection of drug resistant genotypes and the appropriate responses to such selection require detailed knowledge of parasite population structure and genetics. Acquisition of this knowledge for helminth parasites must be given high priority. Therefore, it is important that the genome sequencing resources be applied also to the investigation of parasite population genetic structure, and testing of predicted patterns of population sub-division and gene flow.

Immunology: All helminths across the three taxonomic categories (nematodes, trematodes and cestodes) produce molecules that are able to modulate the host immune responses to support their survival as reproductively active adult worms, and the production of transmission stages that have access to vectors, intermediate hosts, or the environment. However, the mechanisms that initiate and sustain this immune regulation remain incompletely understood. These immunoregulatory mechanisms are important not only in the context of explaining the characteristic chronic infections, the absence of protective immunity after first infection, and the possible development of antiparasitic vaccines, but also for the evaluation of MDA and other treatment programmes. Chemotherapy-based programmes can alter the dynamics of transmission and the burdens of infection in treated communities and are therefore likely to perturb these immunoregulatory relationships. The changes could have unintended consequences for global elimination efforts, such as increased susceptibility to infection (if protective immunity were for instance elicited by established worms that are susceptible to the actions of the drug), or to patency, resulting in increased disease burden in children and/or increased morbidity. Also, the duration of immune responses is unknown and it is difficult to implement immunity-explicit models that could help predict the impact of anthelmintic treatment on immunity parameters.

The unintended immune consequences of treatment are not limited only to the targeted helminth infection; there is increasing evidence of the importance of co-infections, in which parasites and pathogens could interact in a synergistic or antagonistic fashion. Suppressing or removing one parasite species could give selective advantages to others by decreasing immune-mediated competition or inhibitory effects. Possibly as a corollary of phenomena such as these, concurrent helminth infections have been shown to alter optimal vaccine-induced responses, but the consequences of this condition have not been adequately studied, especially in the context of a challenge infection following vaccination. Demands for new and effective vaccines to control other infectious diseases such as tuberculosis, HIV, and malaria, as well as the deployment of vaccines for childhood preventable infections, require a systematic evaluation of confounding factors that may limit vaccine efficacy, including the presence of helminth infections in populations of humans targeted for vaccination.

Not only will interventions have epidemiological effects but also evolutionary implications. In addition to the possible development of anthelmintic resistance already mentioned, any measure that reduces the fitness of the parasite population in terms of its survival, reproduction and transmissibility, will exert some selective pressure, and antiparasitic vaccines will be no exception. Thus, a better understanding of the basic biology of the host-parasite immunological relationship is required to: 1) better understand the likely long-term epidemiological and evolutionary consequences of MDA and any other treatment modality; 2) better manage the immunological impact of helminths, on both helminth and non-helminth infections; and 3) develop helminth vaccines that are safe and effective.

Host-parasite interaction and pathology: In contrast to the view that helminth infections are generally associated with morbidity rather than mortality, the most severe pathology associated with some helminth infections is cancer. Chronic infections with *Op. viverrini* and *C. sinensis*, the Asian liver flukes, have long been associated with cholangiocarcinoma or bile duct cancer. Helminth-associated cancer is, however, not restricted to Asian liver fluke infections. The eggs of *S. haematobium* provoke granulomatous inflammation, ulceration, and pseudopolyposis of the bladder and ureteral walls. Chronic lesions can then evolve into fibrosis, and carcinoma of the bladder (squamous cell carcinoma). All three of these helminth parasites have been designated as Group 1 carcinogens – metazoan parasites that are carcinogenic to humans – by the International Agency for Research on Cancer, WHO. Therefore, not only do these trematodes cause pathogenic helminth infections, but they also are carcinogenic in humans in a similar fashion to several other more well-known biological carcinogens, in particular hepatitis viruses, human papilloma virus and *Helicobacter pylori*. However, there are few studies on the mechanisms of carcinogenesis of these trematode infections. Therefore, the biology of helminth-associated carcinogenesis should be investigated further. In particular, a focus on the components of the host-parasite relationship (including parasite-specific factors) that mediate carcinogenesis is required.

The obligatory *Wolbachia* endosymbiont bacteria in *O. volvulus* and *W. bancrofti* have been implicated in the immune responses and pathogenesis of these filarial infections, including adverse reactions that may follow microfilaricidal and macrofilaricidal treatment. Future studies will help in the further understanding of *Wolbachia*'s role in pathogenesis prior to and after the introduction of MDA.

4.10.3 Vector-filaria and snail-trematode interactions

Very few of the vector-filaria combinations have been characterized in detail, as to geographical distribution, ecological requirements of the insects' aquatic and adult stages, vector competence, vectorial capacity, and local adaptation, among others. Without these studies, detailed mapping of the distribution of vectors and parasites will remain elusive. Vector competence encompasses the processes by which the vectors locate, ingest, and allow the parasites to complete their extrinsic incubation period. For vectors to transmit, not only must they survive such a period but also beyond it (the so-called infective life-expectancy or longevity factor in vector-borne diseases). In general, these processes remain poorly characterized and quantified in those vector-filaria combinations that are responsible for transmission in endemic areas. However, some effort has been spent in doing so for *Simulium-Onchocerca* complexes given the impetus of the OCP and the need to quantify such relationships for their use in mathematical models. Likewise, and in order to explore the likelihood of elimination in LF settings, statistical descriptions of mosquito-*Wuchereria* interactions have received attention. Less is known about natural mosquito-*Brugia*, and tabanid-*Loa* interactions, knowledge of which relies on old descriptive studies that, although still relevant, need to be updated and expanded. Vector competence studies should be complemented by vectorial capacity investigations. Vectorial capacity (a close relative of the basic reproduction ratio in vector-borne diseases) also includes factors such as vector to host ratio, vector biting rate on humans, the propensity of vectors to feed on human or non-human blood hosts, vector mortality, and any seasonal and/or spatial dependencies that may occur in these factors. Knowledge of these, as well as of any density dependence that may operate (e.g. on the density of vectors and/or hosts, on the density of parasites) will inform the design and implementation of vector control and any transmission-blocking intervention that may be developed. Yet knowledge as to if (and how) helminth parasites manipulate these crucial aspects of the interaction is still very scarce;

there is increasing evidence that this is the case in malaria, but experimental and observational studies in filariasis have lagged behind.

Regarding snail-trematode interactions, most efforts have been made for the schistosomes as described above; literature on the ecological, evolutionary, and epidemiological relationships between the other trematodiases referred to in this report and their snail hosts is sparse. It would seem that the reference to 'food-borne trematodiases' (because of the nature of the subsequent intermediate hosts for these parasites) has somewhat decreased the importance of their first, snail hosts. Yet it is within the snail hosts that many important processes allowing the asexual multiplication of the parasite take place. Unlike schistosomes, the eggs of *Clonorchis* and *Opisthorchis* are eaten by the snail hosts (rather than the miracidia locating and invading the snails), but the resulting cercariae also need to find and locate their second intermediate, freshwater fish host. The fish are not just passive transport hosts of the parasites as it is in this host that the metacercariae (the stages infective by digestion of raw, undercooked fish) develop. Therefore, the study of host-trematode interactions for these infections must include those taking place in the snails and the vertebrate intermediate hosts. Difficulties in maintaining the whole life-cycle of these parasites in the laboratory would certainly impose constraints on experimental studies such as those conducted for schistosomes.

5. Intersectoral and cross-cutting issues

5.1 Cross-cutting issues of participation, ownership, empowerment, equity and gender

Effectiveness of control programmes is clearly dependent on a series of interrelated factors that are extremely difficult to orchestrate. Dedicated political commitment is crucial for achieving viable and sustainable interventions even when there is significant support from external funders/donors. In this context, factors such as adequate coverage, education including self-perception of health and illness, community participation, sanitation, compliance, and sustainability are necessary.

Community participation is viewed as the key approach to address helminth infections, improve community health and promote sustainable development in controlling infections; it increases people's autonomy over health care and consequently the empowerment of individuals (463). Unfortunately, most often individuals and communities do not take these diseases seriously because they are unaware of the insidiousness of the cumulative morbidity. Moreover, even when they are aware, still little attention has been given to the communities' interest in actively participating in control programmes and forging relationships between external motivators and community programme officers.

Adopting sound strategies that empower community members to take relatively simple measures to prevent diseases and protect their health, and to adhere to community-directed treatment, is well described in the literature. What is unclear is which strategy is the most effective to address such needs. Most endemic communities lack institutional systems and structures to encourage people to participate in control strategies, and if they are present, they may not function adequately. One example of a successful strategy in neglected tropical disease (NTD) control programmes is the approach used for community-directed treatment with IVM (CDTI) for onchocerciasis control. This approach has evolved into the more general concept of community-directed interventions. A high level of community participation is expected to increase compliance. However, low level of commitment by community leaders, disregard for mass drug distribution (or for the infection at which this is aimed), a greater perceived urgency for the provision of basic needs, and a perception that the programme in question should be the responsibility of the primary health-care system rather than the responsibility of the community, all lead to inadequacies in this approach (464).

Gender differences in health systems and services have been the subject of extensive research, especially with regard to vulnerability to illness, access to treatment, and poverty. Studies have shown variations in terms of life expectancy, risk of morbidity and mortality, health-promoting/seeking behaviours, and use of health-care services. Evidence also shows that different social determinants of health affect gender inequalities in ways that can magnify the impact on health. Most studies on gender have focused mainly on issues affecting women and less on men (*465*).

In human helminthiases, the link between gender and disease has been established through a number of studies especially in onchocerciasis, lymphatic filariasis (LF), and schistosomiasis. These studies have highlighted differences in infection rates (that propagate from childhood into adulthood) which tightly correlate with behavioural differences and occupational activities that determine exposure to vectors/intermediate hosts, social status, access to treatment, and resulting sequelae (*466–471*) similar to those found in leprosy (*472*) and tuberculosis (*39*). The effect of gender and age on socioeconomic status remains poorly understood for the human helminthiases. Little work has been conducted to apply current knowledge from gender studies to the development of gender-related policy and practice across all aspects of the health sector and capacity building. Gender-related health policies should ensure that health systems address gender equity and improve efficiency.

5.2 The impact of global climate change

The effect of global warming on human health has received much interest in recent years (*473*). About 150 000 deaths have occurred and 5 million disability-adjusted life years (DALYs) have been lost annually on a global scale due to climate change over the past 30 years (*474, 475*). It is anticipated that alterations will be triggered in physical and biological systems, inducing shifts in the spatio-temporal distribution of disease vectors and intermediate hosts (*476–479*). However, the precise effects of climate change on vector competence, duration of extrinsic incubation periods, survival of vectors, intermediate hosts and reservoirs, and on transmission cycles in general remain poorly understood for the helminthiases (*480*). It has been postulated that climate change is likely to affect the geographical distribution of freshwater snails, such as *Biomphalaria* spp., the intermediate hosts of S. *mansoni*. An ongoing water resource project, the South-to-North Water Transfer Project, has probably facilitated introduction of the snail intermediate host of S. *japonicum* (*Oncomelania hupensis*) to new potential habitats in northern parts of the People's Republic of China (PRC) due to climate change (*481, 482*).

These ecological and environmental transformations will undoubtedly affect access by human populations to health services, as well as agricultural/husbandry practices. There are two principal strategies for managing or reducing the risks of environmental change: mitigation and adaptation. The former seeks to reduce the presence and strength of anticipated risk factors (when these are known). The latter accepts that some degree of environmental change is inevitable and seeks to limit its negative impacts by encouraging and investing in preparedness. Both strategies require detailed assessment of the existing distribution of the infections, their transmission agents (biological and environmental), and suitable modifications to agricultural and husbandry practices, among others. The combined impact of these determinants on the transmission cycles and rates of exposure to helminth infections of humans is poorly understood. Systematic phenology reviews and experimental investigation will help prioritize models to predict the consequences of climate change on the incidence and severity of human helminthiases. A biology-driven model to assess the potential impact of rising temperature on the transmission of schistosomiasis japonica in the PRC and of long-term temperature changes on the epidemiology and control of intestinal schistosomiasis has been developed (*481, 483, 484*).

5.3 Challenges stemming from environmental and social ecology factors: water-associated diseases and water management

The linkages between water, health and diseases are fundamental to understanding the disease burden in rural communities. On the one hand, water bodies provide breeding sites for disease vectors; on the other, agriculture, aquaculture, and animal husbandry depend on water, and communities need water for consumption and hygiene. The relationships are often bi-directional: water development projects were initially designed to generate hydro-electric power, control flooding, and/or to increase the availability of drinking water and irrigation for agriculture. However, poorly designed systems may enhance the habitats of disease vectors (e.g. of *Anopheles* spp. mosquitoes transmitting malaria and LF, *Simulium* spp. transmitting onchocerciasis, and intermediate host snails transmitting schistosomiasis), disrupt natural hydrological cycles, and impede natural water filtration processes. Some studies have shown that the construction of the Three Gorges Dam in the People's Republic of China (PRC) might have affected the transmission of *S. japonicum* downstream of the dam (*485, 486*). Research needs in this area include acquiring more knowledge on the strengths of interactions between agriculture, water and health in order to carry out specific case studies using integrated applicable solutions that can be appropriately scaled-up. A deeper discussion of these issues will be presented in the reports of DRG6 and the thematic group on Environment, Agriculture and Infectious Diseases (TRG4).

5.4 Limitations in the health services

The success of control programmes can be hampered by the lack of institutional capacity to implement the desired interventions. The acceptability to the population of multiple treatments and the engagement of the community are often overlooked. A study by Massa et al. (*121*) showed that a combined approach of school-based treatment plus community-directed treatment (ComDT) (the latter used by the African Programme for Onchocerciasis Control (APOC) as CDTI) was successful in reducing prevalence and intensity of STHs and schistosomiasis. This process has been subsequently extended to integrated control programmes for many other infectious diseases. ComDT appears to be even more efficient than school-based programmes since it ensures better coverage of especially very young and non-enrolled school-age children. It is important to mention that the ComDT approach may succeed, if well accepted by the communities, as a platform onto which to integrate other interventions (*121*) such as vitamin A supplementation and bednet distribution. Compliance increases the health benefits of integrated interventions and may be more apparent than with single interventions, for which interest wanes over time. The relative merits of these approaches (school-based vs. community-based) depends on the initial endemicity of the infection, the age of the most at-risk groups, and the phase of programme implementation. Encouraging community participation requires investing in continued training of community leaders. Research into the impact of systematic noncompliance on control is needed to address issues of optimal drug delivery to increase compliance (*123–125*).

In disease-endemic countries, access to health services may be limited and existing services deficient. Improvement in this situation should go hand in hand with efforts to control infectious diseases. Evaluation of access to, and utilization of, health services for diagnosis, treatment and surveillance of helminthiases is necessary to help policy-makers develop sustainable programmes, especially in primary health care.

The Health Systems and Implementation Research (TRG3) report shows rightly that activities in the control of infectious diseases form part of the broader health systems actions. The TRG3 report refers to the fact that health systems have a major impact upon, and are affected by, political, economic and social context; they are dynamic entities responding to, among many factors, epidemiological and demographic situations; and finally, they are underpinned by stakeholders and their values. All these points are crucial for the control of infectious diseases including helminth infections.

5.5 Polyparasitism and integration of intervention measures

Polyparasitism is often the norm rather than the exception in poor countries of the tropics and sub-tropics. Studies have demonstrated a positive association between infection intensity and concurrent infection with helminth species, suggesting that individuals with multiple helminthiases may also have the most intense infections (*37–41*). Therefore polyparasitism may have a greater impact on morbidity than the sum of single-species infections. Also, multiple species infections may increase susceptibility to other infections such as malaria or HIV

(*42*, *43*), particularly given the immunosuppresive nature of nematode infections. For example, epidemiological studies in Thailand suggest that elimination of helminth co-infections might increase the frequency of cerebral malaria (*43*, *392*), while in Africa, elimination of helminth co-infections reduced the frequency of acute malaria attacks (*487*, *488*). However, the health impact of polyparasitism has not been studied sufficiently despite its potential significance for public health. Available evidence is typically based on retrospective, secondary analyses of previously collected data, which lack sufficient statistical power and are subject to confounding influences, due to variable socioeconomic or dietary intake factors. It is necessary to investigate the relative impact of single- and multiple-species infections, as well as to evaluate integrated disease control programmes (*44*).

To date, the basis for much of the interaction between worms and malaria is thought to be immunological, with the worms altering the immune response and profoundly affecting the subsequent immune response to malaria infection. However, very few studies (except for schistosomiasis (*489*)) have actually analysed the immune response to worm infection in individuals living in malaria endemic areas, or the actual sequence of infection in areas of different endemicity for the infections concerned. For instance, in highly endemic malaria areas there is a higher chance that infants will acquire malaria prior to helminth infection. This includes very fundamental types of immuno-epidemiological studies, in which, among other things, the humoral and cellular immune responses to crude and defined antigens from different helminth infections are characterized with host age and compared to different levels of malaria parasitaemia and the progression to different levels of clinical malaria. It is clear that further detailed and integrated studies are required to advance our understanding of helminth-malaria interactions and to what extent these can be modulated after mass drug administration (MDA).

Currently available single-drug treatments can simultaneously target as many as four of the helminth neglected tropical diseases, including onchocerciasis, LF, soil-transmitted helminths (STHs), and schistosomiasis. However, more operational research is needed to determine the best implementation strategies for providing these oral drug therapies at a population level; the Global Network for Neglected Tropical Disease Control (GNNTDC) and the World Health Organization (WHO) have started such investigations (*2*, *4*). For example, at-risk populations may be difficult to reach because they live in remote areas or do not attend school; studies are required in the affected regions where resources are limited to identify practical methods to coordinate and execute the proposed treatment plans. Implementation of any helminth control programme at country level will be best developed if strong links are created with already existing interventions, e.g. by adding anthelmintic treatment to well-established vaccination programmes and involving mobile teams that can reach affected populations who live in remote areas without access to routine health care.

The integration of different vertical control programmes may be difficult due to disparities between the population groups who must be targeted for onchocerciasis, LF, STHs, and schistosomiasis control. Studies are necessary to identify optimal and common age groups for integrated control where feasible. There is still the need to face additional political hurdles in order to facilitate cooperation among the different groups working to control the different diseases and fully integrate their activities.

The concept of integrating NTD management should go beyond anthelmintic chemotherapy as the only solution. Longer-term goals should include vaccine development, morbidity control and suppression of transmission of these diseases. The development of better and more sensitive monitoring prior to and after chemotherapy (including those untreated/unvaccinated sections of the population in order to ascertain reductions in environmental transmission and 'herd immunity' benefits), and the improvement of public health measures such as access to clean water, adequate sanitation, improved environmental conditions, housing, and health education are key to integrated management. Another challenge is to address adequately the multi-faceted nature of NTDs, to depart from traditional single disease-centered approaches and adopt a more holistic approach. Substantial efforts are required to perform operational research to implement and evaluate the potential impact of such an approach and to explore the social and socioeconomic structures that contribute to the maintenance of these diseases. The incorporation of pharmacovigilance is necessary, particularly in studying drug combination safety, and optimization of dose rates for antiparasitic efficacy.

6. Regional highlights and research capacity

6.1 Regional highlights

Regions of the world mostly affected by helminthiases include Latin America and the Caribbean Islands, Africa and Asia. Some helminth diseases may be common to most of the endemic regions while others are very specific or may disproportionately affect particular regions. Furthermore, impoverished living conditions and ongoing environmental changes make endemic communities in certain regions more susceptible to more than one infection, resulting in polyparasitism (Figure 1, page 13). These conditions may have an impact on the level of disease endemicity, and on disease progression in different localities. Consequently, there are regional differences in terms of deciding which control and/or other intervention strategies to adopt.

For example, lymphatic filariasis (LF) and/or onchocerciasis are endemic in Africa, tropical areas of the Americas and the Caribbean Islands, and the South-East Asia Region. Where LF is co-endemic with onchocerciasis, ivermectin (IVM) + albendazole (ABZ) is the recommended regimen for intervention; in regions with only LF, diethycarbamazine (DEC) + ABZ is recommended. Where scale-up of mass drug administration (MDA) is required, e.g. for LF control, many of the endemic countries in Africa have adopted the community-directed treatment (ComDT) strategy. This strategy ensures that the community has responsibility for providing treatment to its members, resulting in increased community acceptance and coverage (*490*). However, in India, drug distribution by the health services is the preferred treatment strategy because it is considered less cumbersome and more acceptable than ComDT (*491*). In the Tuvalu Islands, the mass screen and treat (MSAT) strategy has been adopted, in which the entire population is tested and only the infected individuals are treated every 3 months, and retested every 12 months (*492*). Treatment of onchocerciasis is also distinct in different regions. The intervention strategy for the Americas is elimination of the infection reservoir using twice-a-year IVM treatment, and treating all the affected communities in 13 foci within six countries (Brazil, Colombia, Ecuador, Guatemala, Mexico, and Venezuela), whereas in Africa the control strategy has been based on annual IVM treatment only in meso- and hyperendemic regions, for elimination of morbidity.

The human liver flukes (*Op. viverrini*, *Op. felineus* and *C. sinensis*) that cause food-borne trematodiases are an important public health problem, particularly in Asia. People in Thailand, the Lao People's Democratic Republic (Lao PDR), Cambodia and the Socialist Republic of Vietnam are known to be at risk of *Op. viverrini* and *Op. felineus* infection. In South-East Asia, chronic infections with *Op. viverrini* and *C. sinensis* are known to be associated with cholangiocarcinoma, the bile duct cancer (*33*). Clonorchiasis and opisthorchiasis are confined to Asia, while paragonimiasis can be found in Asia, Africa and Latin America. Taeniasis and cysticercosis are endemic in Latin American countries with "hotspots" of the disease in Mexico and several countries in Central America. In the South-East Asian Region, countries like India, Nepal and Bhutan are known to be endemic for *T. solium*. In the Western Pacific Region, taeniasis/cysticercosis is known to be transmitted in the PRC, the Socialist Republic of Vietnam, Cambodia, Lao People's Democratic Republic, the Philippines and Papua New Guinea. The different helminth infections present on the different continents mean that different research capabilities and interventions are required. In the South-East Asian Region, Latin America and Western Pacific Region, various intervention strategies against taeniasis and cysticercosis have been developed (*48, 116*) but none have been adopted in Africa.

6.2 Research capacity

6.2.1 Background

Research capacity relevant to public health is essential for understanding and combating, controlling, and eliminating any disease. This requires appropriate regulatory frameworks, physical infrastructure, investment in human resources, equipment, training, research commitment, institutional support and adequately skilled personnel to design, conduct and publish scientific research (*493*). The level of research capacity varies extensively worldwide, and significant disparities exist between the developed world and developing countries in terms of research and technological expertise and facilities. These differences are mainly due to the major investments made by the developed world in research and development activities, and the proportion of gross domestic product (GDP) that governments are willing to invest in research. In some developed countries, long-term investment has resulted in extensive infrastructure, the existence of national expertise, a tradition in funding, and a more expeditious path between research and implementation of public health policy (e.g. pandemic influenza, bovine tuberculosis, SARS). The ready availability and opportune deployment of such resources has led to rapid advances in controlling infectious agents with epidemic potential. However, in the developing world, and especially in most African countries, investments towards research capacity building to support disease control and elimination efforts are either completely missing or woefully inadequate. There is a paucity of highly trained researchers, and a considerable brain drain of the already insufficient number of trained professionals.

Adequate research capacity for the management of helminthiases and other infectious diseases of poverty forms an essential component of the tools to help meet the millennium development goals (MDGs) (*2, 494*). To achieve these goals, several high-level meetings on research capacity (in Mexico City, Abuja, Accra, Algiers, and more recently Bamako) have called for action though a clear commitment has not yet been made by all participating nations. In Bamako, the Call to Action 2009 urged all stakeholders to "promote and share the discovery and development of, and access to products and technologies addressing neglected and emerging diseases which disproportionately affect low- and middle-income countries". It is evident that more interaction among nations with the same health problems is essential to facilitate exchange of experiences as well as training of individuals to help achieve the MDGs. This requires a great deal of investment from both international and national funding bodies to develop the facilities and the capabilities of researchers, who can drive research aimed at developing more effective tools and strategies to fight the infectious diseases of poverty.

6.2.2 Inequalities in research capacity

Building research capacity is a long-term process that requires a systemic and intersectoral approach to developing appropriate regulatory frameworks, building and maintaining physical infrastructure, and investing in human resources, equipment, and training in a conducive environment of research commitment and institutional support (*493*). Above all, it requires demand for and supply of enhanced scientific research, based on a conviction that research, and particularly health research, can improve the lives of people and spur economic development (here, 'health research' refers to an umbrella term encompassing research in the biomedical, epidemiological, public health, social science and environmental disciplines related to human health). The level of infectious and parasitic diseases research capacity varies greatly across the world, and significant disparities exist in research and technological expertise and facilities between developed and developing countries. Substantial heterogeneity also exists within the latter; in Africa, South Africa (classified as 'scientifically proficient'), and Benin, Egypt, and Mauritius ('scientifically developing') have done reasonably well regarding national investment and productivity in science and technology, with the remaining countries on the continent falling behind ('scientifically lagging countries') (*494*). Inequalities in health research contribute to inequalities in health and ultimately wealth. Some countries, such as Brazil and the People's Republic of China, have made remarkable progress, in part because their governments have invested substantially in health research and capacity building. For science to deliver its promise of improving health and enabling development, all countries should be able to participate equitably in research (*493*).

Inter-country differences are mainly due to the major investments that have been made by the developed world towards research and development (R&D) activities, and to, especially, the proportion of gross domestic product (GDP) that governments are willing to invest in research for an expected return.

In some developed countries, long-term investment has resulted in extensive infrastructure, existence of national expertise and national and international academic prestige, a tradition in research funding, and a more expeditious path between basic and clinical, translational research and its implementation into public health policy and practice. Investment in research and innovative technologies has tremendously improved health in the developed world, because of the clear health research policies, including the setting up of priorities at institutional, national and regional levels. The readily available and opportune deployment of such resources has led to rapid advances in controlling infectious agents that have epidemic potential. However, in the developing world and especially in most African countries, investment in research capacity building to support the prevention, control and elimination of infectious diseases of poverty is insufficient. In addition to the paucity of highly trained researchers, there is a considerable brain drain of the already scarce numbers of trained professionals, fragmentation of research with much duplication of efforts, and a lack of focus on distinct national needs. According to Chauhan (*495*), lack of encouragement, unethical research practices that have left a legacy of mistrust, a colonial past that has left some degree of suspicion and engendered dependency, and most importantly, an environment of political, social, and economic instability, have all contributed to the scarcity of scientific research in Africa. Whatever the reasons for the dearth of research in Africa for Africa, this situation is untenable (*493*) and threatens the long-term sustainability of any disease control programme.

6.2.3 Research capacity in disease-endemic countries

Research must focus on national priorities and high disease burden conditions in disease-endemic countries, with emphasis on evaluating interventions that aim to strengthen research capacity and health systems, and activities that translate knowledge into action and benefits for the local population (*493*). In many countries of Sub-Saharan Africa, Asia, Latin America and the Caribbean, neglected tropical diseases (NTDs) in general, and the helminthiases in particular, inflict a high disease burden (*11, 496–499*). Adequate research capacity for the management of helminthiases and other infectious diseases of poverty, including the NTDs, forms an essential component of the tools needed to meet the MDGs (*500*). Of particular importance is the demonstration of measurable impacts on health, educational success, and economic development, which are essential to convince government officials that financial investment in control programmes generates a tangible, cost-effective return (*501*). It is important that developing countries, supported by developed countries and donors, establish internally competitive national, or regional, research support and training agencies which can prioritize areas of national (regional) interest for potential support, be transparent, and conduct open competitions for the best projects in terms of scientific content and potential impact, possible sustainability, integration of research and training, and leverage of external funding to support the national and regional efforts in research and training.

It is evident that more interaction among nations with common health problems and infectious diseases is essential to facilitate exchange of experience as well as training of individuals to help achieve the MDGs. This requires a great deal of investment from both international and national funding bodies to develop the facilities and the capabilities of scientists who can drive research aimed at developing more effective tools and strategies to fight infectious diseases of poverty. Improving prevention and control strategies for NTDs will result in poverty alleviation and consequent achievement of the MDGs. However, this will require sincere commitment, political resolve, and competitive and transparent mechanisms for using health research as a driver towards sustainable human resource development, economic growth and poverty reduction. Collaborative research is surely one of the best means for strengthening such research capacity, and in general, it has been the case that scientists in disease-endemic countries welcome collaboration with the more industrialized nations of the so-called 'North' as a vehicle for overcoming barriers to conducting research, obtaining training and funding, and promoting the exchange of ideas. Unfortunately, scientists of disease-endemic countries seem less enthusiastic about collaborating with countries from their own continents and regions (*493*). In part, this is because research funding opportunities for such South–South collaboration have been limited (but see below for a number of Brazil–Africa initiatives).

It is also true that most efforts towards health research and NTD capacity building in disease-endemic countries have been made on the impulse of institutions based in industrialized countries. A major international organization that has played an important role in building research capacity is the Special Programme for Research and Training in Tropical Diseases (TDR) of the World Health Organization (WHO). This programme has, over the past 30 years, sponsored the training of graduates from disease-endemic countries at both master's and doctorate levels, as well as specialist technological training, and has provided further support (in the form of re-entry grants) for graduates to return to their own countries and establish productive research. The emphasis is on developing the research, management and leadership capacities of scientists in disease-endemic countries, fostering research environments for long-term sustainability, quality processes and strategic partnerships (http://apps.who.int/tdr/svc/grants/calls/grants-dec-investigators-2010). More recently, in 2010, TDR has sponsored exchange of research and training between African scientists from Niger, Nigeria, and Uganda and the National Institute of Parasitic Diseases, Chinese Center for Disease Control and Prevention in Shanghai regarding schistosomiasis control. This has resulted in a fruitful South–South connection between two previously separate TDR-supported networks in schistosomiasis, namely, the Regional Network for Asian Schistosomiasis and other Zoonotic

Helminths (RNAS+) and the Regional Network for Schistosomiasis in Africa (RNSA). Through this newly cemented collaboration, the two networks can learn from one another to build their capacity and expertise (http://apps.who.int/tdr/svc/publications/tdrnews/issue-86/schisto-control). Another significant step in the right direction is the proposed relocation to Africa of the TDR-supported Initiative to Strengthen Health Research Capacity in Africa (ISHReCA), at present based at WHO/TDR in Geneva, and sponsored by the Wellcome Trust among other funders (http://www.who.int/tdr/partnerships/initiatives/ishreca/en/).

In 2009, the Wellcome Trust funded the African Institutions Initiative, aiming to develop institutional capacity to support and conduct health-related research vital to enhancing people's health, lives and livelihoods through the formation of seven new international and pan-African consortia with each partnership being led by an African institution (http://www.wellcome.ac.uk/News/Media-office/Press-releases/2009/WTX055742.htm). This is in addition to longer-established African-based programmes such as the KEMRI-Wellcome Trust Research Programme at the Centre of Geographical Medicine Research Coast (CGMRC), in Kilifi, Kenya (http://www.kemri-wellcome.org/). There are many other such programmes and examples of current capacity building initiatives in the area of health research and NTDs, particularly in Africa, which have external support. The African Capacity Building Foundation (ACBF), though not focused on health, aims at building sustainable human and institutional capacity for poverty reduction in Africa. Since its inception in 1991, 20 years ago, the ACBF has supported a total of 246 programmes and projects in some 44 Sub-Saharan African countries and committed more than US$ 400 million to capacity building (http://www.acbf-pact.org/).

Regarding South–South initiatives, Brazil has, since 2008, supported collaboration and training of African scientists through the Pro-Africa Program for Thematic Cooperation in Science and Technology of the National Research Council (CNPq, http://www.cnpq.br). This scheme funds meetings, research and seed money to evaluate the potential of collaborative efforts. In partnership with TWAS (the Academy of Sciences for the Developing World, http://www.twas.org/), an autonomous international organization based in Italy that promotes scientific capacity and excellence for sustainable development in the South, CNPq also supports students from African countries to be trained in Brazil at postgraduate and postdoctoral levels. Furthermore, the Oswaldo Cruz Foundation (FIOCRUZ), with support from the Brazilian government, recently established an initiative with the Mozambican National Institute of Health to create a master's programme in health sciences, with the goal of providing qualified human resources for health research and innovation for Mozambique (*502*). For a more comprehensive account of Brazil's conception of South–South cooperation in health see (*503*).

6.2.4 Challenges for research capacity building in disease-endemic countries

Research and development investment in the areas of NTDs in general and helminthiases in particular pales into insignificance (*499*) in comparison to that for HIV/AIDS, malaria and tuberculosis (TB) according to the G-FINDER reports of 2009 (*504*) and 2010 (http://www.policycures.org/downloads/g-finder_2010.pdf). It is therefore not surprising, given the overall shrinking levels of R&D investment made in helminthiases by industrialized nations (*499*), that in most disease-endemic countries, research on NTDs and helminthiases is not considered a priority, receives very little attention and is further hindered by some of the obstacles described below.

Outflow of trained staff: The science and health sectors in Africa, and to a lesser extent Latin America and parts of Asia, suffer from a continuous outward drain of trained staff, a problem that donors have addressed primarily by financing training. But training is only part of the solution to building human capacity, because low salaries, poor and unattractive working conditions and environments, and lack of institutional incentives to allow the development of individuals' full scientific potential in their own countries also contribute to low morale and high outflow. Technical assistance and training have often proved ineffective in helping to build sustained capacity. What is needed is a comprehensive approach to human resource management as well as a systemic approach to capacity building (*505*), including recognition of the importance of developing a strong research culture in disease-endemic countries.

Lack of governmental support: A report commissioned by the World Bank showed that with the exception of South Africa, Egypt and a few others, most disease-endemic countries in Africa (and also in Latin America with the exception of Brazil and Cuba, and in Asia, excepting the PRC and India) incur very low national investments in research in general, and have low productivity in science and technology (*494*). This generalization probably masks the fact that scientifically less advanced countries may have reasonable capacity in certain areas, but there is no doubt that the situation of health research in Africa is dire (*493*). Another World Bank report (*505*) found that most capacity support remains fragmented, that the countries do not fully "own" the capacity building agenda, and that the challenges of capacity building vary across sectors within countries as well as across countries. Research capacity building requires the investment of meaningful amounts of funds which many of the governments of disease-endemic countries are not willing to make available because research is considered as a long-term undertaking that only rich countries can afford, and because of other perceived pressing needs. Governments are inclined to follow agendas demanded by powerful, well-organized lobby interests more readily than those sought by seemingly weaker or more diffuse, decentralized interests, such as investment in education and health (*505*). There is lack of sufficient funds from individual governments of disease-endemic countries to support institutional infrastructure, to fund medium- and long-term research projects, and to create well-remunerated job opportunities for local scientists; these are major factors which prevent African scholars trained abroad from returning to their home countries to pursue careers in health research. Despite the small national inputs, research capacity development has been identified as an important endeavour that should be fostered in order to obtain the evidence-based knowledge that is relevant to the health concerns of local communities and that policy-makers can use for implementation of adequate practices (*506*).

Shortages in basic and operations research and specialized training: The successes achieved by control programmes, like the former Onchocerciasis Control Programme in West Africa (OCP), the current African Programme for Onchocerciasis Control (APOC), and the Schistosomiasis Control Initiative (SCI), have been partly realized because of the fundamental and operations research carried out within the umbrella of programme activities (*500*). In most disease-endemic countries there is moderate capacity for research in the areas of epidemiology, parasitology, malacology, and entomology, but research capacity is lacking or dwindling in other specialized areas that are essential to support successful control measures, such as transmission dynamics modelling and advanced statistical analysis of helminth and NTD epidemiological data, parasite population biology and genetics, vector ecology, and detection and monitoring of resistance to anti-parasitic drugs and anti-vectorial measures. Expertise in these areas and evidence-based research output are essential for supporting appropriate decisions by policy-makers in the context of implementation and evaluation over time of single and/or integrated helminth control programmes (*499, 507*). (In this context, authors of this report (MYO-A, RKP, M-GB) recently organized and taught a course, funded by the Leverhulme–Royal Society Africa Award, on "Epidemiology, transmission dynamics and control of vector-borne and neglected tropical diseases" at the University of Ghana, including topics on anthelmintic resistance, vector biology, infectious disease modelling, and NTD epidemiology and control.)

Insufficient mentorship: In many disease-endemic countries, scientists and/or lecturers from research institutions and universities work mainly as individuals rather than as teams. This leaves the new entrant, the young scientist/lecturer, in a place where there is little or no guidance, direction or environment to facilitate his/her career development and progression. Moreover, facilities and inputs for scientific research available to the young scientist are limited. To facilitate research capacity in disease-endemic countries, there is a need for senior scientists/faculty staff members to mentor junior researchers. Having a mentor with expertise, peer esteem, and networking skills provides an invaluable triad function: guidance and direction for the development of a career pathway; research facilities, laboratories, and group support for practical experience; and access to a network of contacts for projection in the national and international arenas. Mentors and role models provide not only exposure to robust and demanding academic and research environments and a vision of what is expected and possible to achieve, but also opportunities to participate and present in international conferences, and obtain feedback on research dissemination activities, manuscripts, oral presentations, and grant preparation. The introduction of junior fellowships by the European Foundation Initiative for African Research into Neglected Tropical Diseases (EFINTDs) is a step in the right direction, as young scientists will receive mentorship from experienced scientists at strong research institutions in both the North and South. This should help raise a generation of scientists with the required expertise to serve as mentors for the next generation. Mentorship programmes are crucial in disease-endemic countries, since unlike the institutions of developed nations, most disease-endemic countries do not have opportunities for post-doctoral internship and further training that new PhD graduates often have access to in the North. It will be very helpful to disease-endemic countries if international funding agencies were able to provide more fellowships with mentorship options for promising junior scientists, just after completing their PhDs, who are willing to remain in or return to their home countries to build their own careers with the intention of focusing on their countries' research needs (508).

Incomplete access to literature and unedited databases: Strict open access publication policies and subsidies by the research funders of wealthier nations, and the growth of prestigious and high impact open access journals (for instance in the Public Library of Science and BioMed Central families) have ameliorated the access of scientists in disease-endemic countries to high quality and updated peer-reviewed research. In particular, BioMed Central has recently launched "Open Access Africa", a collection of initiatives designed to increase the output and visibility of scientific research published by African learning institutes. The Kwame Nkrumah University of Science and Technology (KNUST) in Kumasi, Ghana, was the first African Foundation Member to participate in BioMed Central's free membership scheme (http://www.biomedcentral.com/developingcountries/events/openaccessafrica). However, a considerable amount of investment by higher education and research institutions is needed to maintain the necessary funding for electronic journals, digitized archives, bibliographic databases, and printed literature that are not easily available in disease-endemic countries. Furthermore, good internet access is sometimes lacking in disease-endemic countries, which in turn limits the access of researchers in those countries to open access information via the internet. For a compilation of web-based bibliography databases of epidemiology, parasitology and tropical medicine resources from the Spanish-speaking Latin America and Caribbean regions see (24). Without affiliation to a strong library in an academic institution, individual internet access even at broadband speed is not sufficient. This hampers research and research capacity. As a positive example, the Brazilian Federal Agency for the Support and Evaluation of Graduate Education (CAPES) subscribes to all major peer-review journals, a remarkable effort to make scientific publications available to all academic and educational institutions in Brazil. In addition, CAPES works with the Cambridge Overseas Trust to offer the CAPES Cambridge Scholarship, which welcomed its first recipients (Brazilian nationals) for PhD training in October 2011 (http://www.cambridgetrusts.org/partners/capes-brazil.html).

The issue of open access to helminth epidemiology databases for the purposes of mathematical modelling is more fully discussed in (507). This ongoing issue has been an important hurdle in developing collaborative programmes and was addressed in the preparatory meetings for the Bamako Call to Action (509). While several institutions would like to have all the data collected from countries where diseases of the poor are prevalent placed on open access databases, this proposal has not had general acceptance because the data have been generated, at great cost, by low- and middle-income countries yet appear to give countries with highly-structured efficient institutions access to the data at apparently no cost. Analysis of these data should be shared between low- and middle-income countries before being open to others, or password-protected access could be granted after mutually beneficial agreements or memoranda of understanding for joint analysis and publication of hard-earned data have been signed by participating institutions and researchers (509). Intellectual property issues are also in need of further discussion (510, 511). Investment in data collection and curation can be substantial, and there has been little mutual collaboration between the developed countries of the North using data from developing countries of the South. It is clear that capacity building for data analysis and translation of findings for improving health, as well as new research questions to be addressed, need further discussion. A system needs to be developed where different stakeholders will participate and share findings (509).

Lack of advanced enabling technology tools: Disease-endemic countries face challenges in research capacity for helminthiases and other infectious diseases, especially in areas that require the application of advanced technology for disease control such as functional genomics and bioinformatics research. Reasons for this include lack of trained personnel in such specialized areas, lack of appropriate infrastructure and equipment, and the brain drain of the few local scientists and health professionals who do have the expertise. Research capacity building in disease-endemic countries faces the greatest challenge in areas requiring the application of advanced technologies such as genetics for disease control, genomics, functional genomics (and other 'omics'), bioinformatics and computational biology, that can, in the medium and long terms, have a major impact on disease control or elimination (512, 513). There is a lack of expertise in disease-endemic countries for the development of new reagents, products and approaches for diagnosis, anthelmintics, vaccines, and integrated vector control, which are crucial for the sustained success of current programmes for control and elimination of helminthiases (*514*). If disease-endemic countries had adequate research capacity to develop effective functional genomics tools and bioinformatics, areas like the study of gene function could be applied to develop novel drugs, for instance based on local natural products.

The path forward is not impossible, however. Some disease-endemic countries in South America, the Caribbean and the African regions, despite similar challenges, have been able to develop adequate research capacity. For example, Brazil, Cuba and South Africa have made major technological advancements in the field of functional genomics, bioinformatics and vaccine development. Notably, the scientific output and impact of these countries' researchers have increased internationally, and consequently the brain drain has been reduced or halted (*47*). Such progress is mostly due to the financial investments made by governments to build and support adequate research capacity in their national institutions. This is now yielding expertise in new technologies, leading to the development of innovative interventions and effective management of various diseases, with resultant progress in infectious disease control. For instance, the first effective meningitis B vaccine was developed at the Cuban Finlay Institute (http://www.finlay.sld.cu/english/eindex.htm), and was recently licensed to GlaxoSmithKline (*515*). The FIOCRUZ/Bio-Manguinhos and Butantan Institutes of Brazil and other collaborative institutions are full members in the product development partnerships (PDPs) of the Human Hookworm Vaccine Initiative (*516*). The PRC is one of the world's leading producers of penicillin; and the PRC, India and Brazil produce praziquantel for schistosomiasis treatment. The National Institute of Parasitic Diseases, Chinese Center for Disease Control and Prevention in Shanghai, following a collaborative effort between Chinese, European and African scientists, has investigated the effects of artemether, singly or in combination with praziquantel, against the major human schistosome species (*517*). The Serum Institute of India is the world's leading manufacturer of diphtheria-pertussis-tetanus vaccine. Over 60% of the United Nations Children's Fund vaccine requirements for the Expanded Programme on Immunization are met by Brazil, Cuba, India, and Indonesia (*518*).

6.2.5 National, regional, and global efforts and strategies towards capacity building for research in infectious diseases of poverty

North–South partnerships: Given the lack of political will and financial commitment by most disease-endemic countries to support research capacity building, the role of global and regional efforts has become crucial in supporting and sustaining the control of helminth infections. These efforts include various established research partnerships between developed countries and developing nations. Establishing these North–South partnerships in the form of consortia, networks and collaborations between research institutions has made valuable contributions to research capacity and should be encouraged, although it requires significant financial investment (*46, 47, 519*). These partnerships are essential for the training of skilled personnel in research methods and dissemination, the translation of results of research into tangible actions, products, or improved practices and policies for the benefit of communities and individuals (*47, 520, 521*), and the deployment of current interventions or the development of novel strategies within national, regional, and global control programmes (*519*).

For such partnerships to work effectively, they should include major players such as local research institutions, universities, researchers of infectious disease of poverty, managers of control programmes, and policy-makers. They should also provide a forum for active involvement of the disease-endemic countries and their scientists to ensure that the priority needs of these countries including the training of local human resources are met. For a more comprehensive account of 'desirables' in establishing 'win-win' partnerships between the North and the South, readers are referred to the '11 principles for research in partnership with developing countries' prepared and published by the Swiss Commission for Research Partnerships with Developing Countries (KFPE) (*522*)(*42*), more recently extended to 12 principles (*523, 524*). Bonfoh et al. (*521*) discuss how the application of these principles, and the evolution of the partnerships from a very basic field station driven by external projects to a fully-fleshed research centre partnered with other African institutions, ensured that research at the Swiss Centre for Scientific Research (CSRS) in Côte d'Ivoire survived a decade of serious civil unrest.

Malaria research initiatives are good examples of integrated success. Although it is a large and highly competitive field, a number of networks exist to foster collaboration, communication, and interactions not only amongst international members but also among local members. An example is the Biology and Pathology of Malaria Parasite (BioMalPar), a network of excellence funded by the European Commission, which has been successful in establishing and strengthening malaria communities and laboratories in both Europe and malaria-endemic countries (*525*). A more recent example is the creation of the International Centers of Excellence for Malaria Research (ICEMR), which has established a global network of independent research centres in malaria-endemic settings to provide knowledge, tools, and evidence-based strategies to support researchers working in a variety of endemic areas, especially within government and health-care institutions.

South–South partnerships: In addition to North–South partnerships, research capacity building can be reinforced by facilitating and providing more opportunities for South–South collaborations (*502, 503*). For instance, in the Latin American and Caribbean region, Brazil and Cuba have made major research investments resulting in a calibre of research expertise and research institutions that are recognized internationally (*503, 515*). These well-established institutions could play a major role as regional and inter-continental focal points for South–South collaborations and capacity strengthening for other endemic countries, such as the above mentioned Brazil–Africa programmes (*502, 503*). In Africa, only a few countries, such as South Africa, have developed sound fiscal policies supporting knowledge-based development and leading to wealth creation. This has enabled them to invest in science and technology, build substantial research capacity (*494*), and importantly, to provide attractive remuneration packages to keep their scientists and other expertise in the country. With such expertise and infrastructure, South Africa could also serve as a regional focal point for South–South collaborations within Africa and between other disease-endemic countries.

Since such partnerships involve considerable financial commitment, extended and continued support will still be needed from global and regional donors, including the WHO/TDR and other major agencies, schemes, research and development institutions and funding bodies committed to capacity building such as: the Health Programme of the European Commission (http://ec.europa.eu/health/programme/funding_schemes/index_en.htm); the training and capacity building programmes of the Parasitology, Health and Development Section (SPHD) of the former Danish Bilharziasis Laboratory (now DBL–Institute for Health Research and Development (http://www.ivs.life.ku.dk/English/Sections/SPHD.aspx)), and of the former Swiss Tropical Institute (now Swiss Tropical and Public Health Institute (Swiss TPH) at Basel (http://www.swisstph.ch/)); the US Agency for International Development (USAID) (http://www.usaid.gov/), and in particular the USAID's Neglected Tropical Disease Program (http://www.neglecteddiseases.gov/index.html); the Neglected and Other Infectious Diseases Program of the B&MGF (http://www.gatesfoundation.org/topics/Pages/neglected-diseases.aspx); the New York-based Ford Foundation International Fellowships Program (http://www.fordifp.net/); the International Development Research Centre of Canada, IDRC (http://www.idrc.ca); AusAID (http://www.ausaid.gov.au/) in Australia; the Institut de Recherche pour le Développement, IRD (http://www.ird.fr/) in France; the Department for International Development of the UK, DFID (http://www.dfid.gov.uk/); the Wellcome Trust (http://www.wellcome.ac.uk/), and the Medical Research Council, MRC (http://www.mrc.ac.uk/index.htm) also in the UK, as well as other foundations, initiatives and programmes (*526*) which also provide awards to support candidates from disease-endemic countries for postgraduate studies at master's and doctoral levels, post-doctoral careers, and research projects. However, these funding opportunities are highly competitive and therefore for nationals of disease-endemic countries to access such funds, local scientists should establish strong networks and collaborations and also strengthen their publication and proposal-writing skills to enable them to tap into such opportunities for research capacity building (*508*).

An important need to be addressed by both North–South and South–South partnerships is that of improving the graduate-level training for students in disease-endemic countries. Unfortunately, the NTD knowledge base in disease-endemic countries is often not extensive and the investigators who are involved in intervention programmes are usually associated with ministries of health rather than with national universities. Although this still would entail a great deal of involvement by partners from the North, if external universities could provide support for investigators to provide in-country training within disease-endemic countries to build up a critical mass of able personnel, the ability to carry out and evaluate NTD control without relying on external direction will one day become a reality. Often, for good training, disease-endemic countries students must travel elsewhere, which contributes to the exit of qualified scientists who stay in their country of training rather than returning to their home countries.

In conclusion, support for and from disease-endemic countries for building relevant, disease-endemic country-led research capacity for the control and elimination of human helminthiases and infectious diseases of poverty is still inadequate despite the many initiatives that exist, as these initiatives mainly focus on research portfolios, researcher profiles, and administrative requirements of the developed world, despite the best of intentions (*508*, *527*). Thus a large proportion of the funding for building research capacity in disease-endemic countries has tended to originate from donor agencies, funding bodies, and research institutions whose epicentre is not located in disease-endemic countries, and whose principal investigators and research leaders represent the interests of academic centres from the North rather than those from the South. This requires a concerted effort by the disease-endemic countries and the many national, regional, and global initiatives towards the development of true 'win-win' partnerships. This would be a welcome path towards meeting the MDGs.

7. Regional and national policies on research and their implications

7.1 Background

Improving prevention and control strategies for neglected tropical diseases (NTDs) and helminthiases in particular will result in poverty alleviation and consequently achievement of the millennium development goals (MDGs). However, it requires sincere commitment and governmental political resolve to use health research as a driver towards sustainable human resources development, economic growth and poverty reduction. Innovative technologies and investment in research have tremendously improved health in the developed world because of the clear health research policies, including the setting up of priorities at regional, national and institutional levels. In most developing countries however, because there are no clear policies on health research to drive research efforts, research is fragmented, with duplication of effort and lack of focus on distinct national needs. Intensified efforts and cooperation between researchers, government agencies and policy-makers are therefore required in disease-endemic countries to develop strategies that support short- and long-term research efforts for NTDs and helminthiases in particular. Such efforts should be aimed at providing evidence for health-related actions and practice in general, at reducing health inequalities, and in particular at addressing the health needs of the poorer segments of the populations.

7.2 Regional health research policies

The African governments have recognized the importance of adopting sound policies on health research and the potential implications that such policies may have for fostering population health in particular and national development more generally. Consequently, several high-level meetings on health research and policy have taken place recently (mentioned in section 6.2.1); their emphasis has been on policy formulation for the shaping and strengthening of health research and the facilitation and implementation of research strategies to support national progress towards controlling infectious diseases of poverty within their own countries and thus towards economic growth. At the Heads of State and Governments of the Organization of African Unity (OAU) summit held in Abuja, Nigeria, April 2001, the focus was on addressing exceptional challenges of HIV/AIDS, tuberculosis and other related infectious diseases (now NTDs) including helminthiases. The Abuja declaration in 2001 called for action for the development of new and more appropriate policies on health research, practical strategies, effective implementation mechanisms and concrete monitoring structures to ensure adequate and effective control of the diseases (*528*).

The Algiers declaration in 2008 by the African Regional Ministerial Conference on Research for Health aimed at narrowing the knowledge gap to improve Africa's health. The ministers of health recognized the various challenges confronting the health of their peoples and committed to implement strategies and policy on health research at both regional and national levels, aiming to: 1) develop and strengthen adequate national health research policies and strategic frameworks based on national health research and knowledge systems; and 2) create or strengthen South–South and North–South cooperation including technology transfer, and support research capacity building (529). Also, at the Bamako Call to Action in 2008 on Research for Health by ministers and representatives of ministries of health, science and technology, education, foreign affairs, and international cooperation from 53 countries, the focus was on developing and strengthening policies on health research and innovation for health, and development of equity at the national and regional levels. At these 2008 meetings, another important theme was the need for financial investment in health research by all governments of Africa, including a pledge for the allocation of at least 2% of national health expenditure, and at least 5% of external aid for health projects and programmes for research and research capacity building (530).

The purpose of developing these policies and strategies for health research at both the regional and national levels is to ensure that all the necessary resources are available for quality and innovative research that can translate into improving the health of the populations and subsequently into economic growth. There is a strong linkage between health improvements, poverty reduction, and long-term economic growth, as well as a vicious circle, in that disease burden slows down the productivity and economic growth that are needed to solve the health problems. Thus improvement in health at national levels would translate into higher socioeconomic development, leading to progress towards meeting the MDGs.

7.3 National health research policies

Despite the various high-level meetings on health research and the calls for action in Abuja, Accra, Algiers and Bamako, a clear commitment has not yet been made by all participating nations. Some African countries, and South Africa in particular, have been responsive to policy demands on health research funding (494), whilst many other countries are yet to meet the recommended national government budget allocation for research funding. It has been recommended by the Commission on Health Research for Development that at least 2% of national health budgets and at least 5% of development aid should be invested in health research and on research capacity building. More research outcomes can be expected if an upward adjustment is made in the overall research budget. Such gains have been demonstrated by some disease-endemic countries, such as Brazil (*531*). Policy-makers must also ensure that research is enhanced by increased financial and political support (*532*).

7.4 Recommendations

Some policies on health research have already been developed and implemented at both national and regional levels in the African, South American and Caribbean Island, and the South-East Asian regions. However, more policies are needed to ensure that all the necessary resources are available for quality and innovative research that can translate into improving the health of the people and economic growth. It is therefore recommended that:

- Member States of the African, American (Latin America and Caribbean Islands), and South-East Asia Regions promote and support the development of regional policies on health. Policies supporting the development of effective linkages and partnerships with international health research agencies are necessary to augment regional health research capability.

- Regional commitment and strong advocacy be put in place to strengthen policies on health research aimed at providing evidence to justify health actions and practices. These policies must be flexible and responsive to the short- and long-term national needs. Cooperation and active interaction among Member States will facilitate the development of clear policies in the countries and institutions that will enhance research capacity building and networking towards equitable health development.

- African countries put in place research-friendly legislative reforms that facilitate exchange of expertise and data whilst ensuring protection of intellectual property rights. Strong and long-standing advocacy is needed to encourage policy-makers to ensure that more financial and political will is extended towards scientific research.

- The regional and national innovation sector emphasizes the development of comprehensive policies and strategies for supervision across all sectors. This approach gives attention to transparency in terms of funding and its disbursement, strategic planning, priority-setting, knowledge management and demand creation (*533*).

8. Research priority recommendations to policy and decision-makers

Successful intervention against human helminthiases depends on optimal utilization of available control measures and development of new tools and strategies. Currently, many of the ongoing anthelmintic control programmes are based on annual mass drug administration (MDA). The expenditure on delivery of programmes to administer anthelmintic chemotherapy has resulted in millions of infected or exposed people being treated for these infections, with likely significant health benefits. However, the development of diagnostic techniques and strategies for epidemiological monitoring and evaluation (M&E), as well as the application of mathematical and statistical methods to inform control efforts from a programmatic perspective, has somewhat lagged behind these laudable initiatives. The research agenda has been fragmented, lacking a systematic focus on critical issues.

The key drivers of present and future patterns of human helminthiases, as well as the determinants of success in controlling such infections, are often environmental and social in nature, making it necessary to use an intersectoral approach for control. This approach will include not only drug distribution, but also environmental components such as improvement of sanitation and drainage, access to clean water, adequate excreta disposal and solid waste removal, access to health services for diagnosis and treatment, adequate housing and health education. Moreover, the health impact of polyparasitism is significant for public health and is certainly a challenge for the development of control programmes. Inadequate coverage and sustainability of programmes makes the implementation of control/elimination of helminthiases in endemic countries difficult. Additionally, few mathematical models have been effectively used to support decisions in the context of the implementation and evaluation of helminth control programmes in real time, and their full potential to aid control/elimination efforts has yet to be realized.

Solutions to the research gaps and priorities identified in this report are dependent upon knowledge of the relevant and fundamental parasite biology. In this context, it is of serious concern that current interventions are based on the application of old research. This is best illustrated by the reliance on single or very few drugs, most of which have been in use for many years (decades in some cases), and none of which are efficacious in all settings, as well as by the use of often insensitive diagnostic tests that are in some cases older than the drugs.

In view of all this, and for each of the five umbrella areas highlighted by DRG4 members, the group agreed on the following recommendations as priority research areas that would enable advances in the field of helminthiasis control and identification of the novel tools required for elimination of the public health problem posed by these infections or their reservoirs.

8.1 Intervention

While MDA has logistical advantages and seems to have worked well in morbidity reduction programmes based on preventative chemotherapy (e.g. schistosomiasis, onchocerciasis), annual distribution may not necessarily be optimal to achieve transmission control or local elimination of infection, and increased frequency may be necessary. By the same token, it may be necessary to decrease treatment frequency in areas of low transmission according to cost–effectiveness studies. Therefore, research is needed to:

- Optimize the deployment of existing intervention tools to maximize impact (including impact against polyparasitism) and sustainability. The tools include pharmaceuticals, vaccines, vector control and ecohealth approaches (sanitation, clean water, improved nutrition, education). Sustainability depends on minimizing selection for drug resistance and maintaining community support.
- Develop novel control tools to improve impact and sustainability. The tools include pharmaceuticals, vaccines, vector control and ecohealth approaches and how to deliver them optimally and cost effectively.
- Whenever possible, steer intervention from disease control towards permanent elimination.

8.2 Epidemiology and surveillance

The development of adequate techniques for diagnosis and surveillance of helminth infections is crucial to the successful control of these important neglected infectious diseases. In particular, it is essential to:

- Improve available diagnostic tests, specifically their sensitivity and specificity (ability to diagnose infection at low prevalence in elimination settings and confirm cure/absence of infection), multiplex capacity, and ability to measure infection intensity and detect drug resistance.
- Develop new diagnostic tests using biomarkers of infection that reflect infection intensity.
- Standardize and validate methodologies and protocols for diagnosis in M&E settings.
- Develop and validate clinical, phenotypic and molecular methods for monitoring of drug efficacy and resistance.
- Develop and validate questionnaire-based methods for diagnosis of helminth infections.
- Link measures of diagnostic performance for the tests optimized or developed in (2) and (3) above with statistical/mathematical tools to support monitoring and evaluation of helminth control programmes.

8.3 Environment and social ecology

Despite considerable recent advances in the epidemiological understanding of polyparasitism and the recognition by various funding agencies of the importance of conducting multi- and interdisciplinary research on the environmental and social ecology of infectious diseases, our understanding of the public health impact of polyparasitism is still inadequate and will necessitate to:

- Identify the social and environmental structures that contribute to the maintenance of helminth infection (including polyparasitism) for developing multi-disciplinary interventions.
- Develop maps of helminth infection and co-infection as well as of intermediate hosts' and vectors' distribution to enable accurate assessment of distribution and burden of disease.
- Develop strategies incorporating delivery of multiple interventions at various levels to maximize sustainability of control programmes in general and of integrated NTD control in particular.
- Assess the contribution of systematic non-compliant persons as well as of migrants and refugees, pregnant/lactating women and under five-year olds to the maintenance of transmission.
- Develop strategies (taking gender issues into account) to increase community participation, awareness of ill-health processes, ownership and empowerment, as well as equity in access by communities and risk groups to health services.
- Identify and evaluate climate and environmental changes that impact helminth infections.

8.4 Data and modelling

To realize the full potential of policy-relevant models and helminth modelling studies in general, it will be necessary to:

- Develop and refine models to investigate relationships between infection and morbidities to aid programmes aiming to reduce the burden of disease (elimination of public health problem). Such models need to take into account cumulative effects of chronic disease for evaluation of disease burden and the impact on such burden of control interventions.
- Develop and refine models to investigate relationships between infection and transmission thresholds to aid programmes aiming to eliminate the infection reservoir. Such models should determine end-points from programmatic viewpoints, integrating models with data to

determine reinfection rates, changes in the force of infection, optimal treatment frequencies, and the dynamics of transmission breakpoints for the host-parasite combinations prevailing in endemic areas.
- Increase the use and application of epidemiological models to aid M&E and surveillance, the design of cost-effective sampling protocols and the monitoring of intervention efficacy including drug resistance. These models should be linked to cost-effectiveness analyses of the interventions and their alternatives.
- Develop metapopulation and spatially-explicit parasite transmission models.
- Develop and validate mathematical models for co-infections.
- Develop models for investigation of climate change on helminth infections and their control.

8.5 Biology research

It is our contention that there is a lack of investment in strategic basic helminth biology research. Development of a new generation of more effective interventions will only happen if there is a significant new long-term investment in such strategic research that should aim to:

- Investigate how helminth parasites modulate host–parasite interactions at the population and within-host levels, including the impact on the host immune response of concurrent infection with other helminth and non-helminth pathogens, the impact of parasite control interventions on such host–parasite interactions, and how concurrent infections affect clinical outcomes and the host's ability to seroconvert upon vaccination.
- Define the determinants and mechanisms of helminth-induced pathologies, including carcinogenesis, and excess human mortality.
- Identify the mechanisms of host immune responses to helminths, and translate knowledge of these mechanisms into rational strategies for vaccine development.
- Annotate parasite genomes and transcriptomes and develop tools for parasite functional genomics in key species.
- Define parasite (and vector/intermediate host) population and ecological genetic structures in the contexts of genetic responses to interventions within and between parasite populations, parasite transmission, and epidemiology.

9. Conclusions

Using the prioritization process described in Chapter 2, the top ten research priorities for helminth infections are:

1. Research to optimize the deployment of existing intervention tools to maximize impact (including against polyparasitism) and sustainability. The tools include pharmaceuticals, vaccines, vector control and ecohealth approaches (sanitation, clean water, improved nutrition and education). Sustainability depends on minimizing selection for drug resistance and maintaining community support.
2. Research to develop novel control tools which will improve impact and sustainability. The tools include pharmaceuticals, vaccines, vector control and ecohealth approaches and how to deliver them optimally and cost effectively.
3. Research to improve available diagnostic tests, specifically their sensitivity, specificity, multiplex capacity, and ability to measure infection intensity, and detect drug resistance. Sensitivity and specificity are mostly important to enable diagnosis of infection at low prevalence in elimination settings and to confirm cure/absence of infection.
4. Research to standardize and validate methodologies and cost-effective protocols for diagnosis in monitoring and evaluation (M&E) settings.
5. Research to develop strategies incorporating delivery of multiple interventions at various levels to maximize sustainability of control programmes in general and integrated NTD control in particular.
6. Research to develop strategies (taking gender issues into account) to increase: awareness of ill-health processes, community participation, ownership and empowerment, as well as equity in access by communities and risk groups to health services.
7. Research to develop and refine models to investigate the relationships between infection and morbidities to aid programmes aiming to reduce the burden of disease (elimination of public health problem). Such models need to take into account the cumulative effects of chronic disease for evaluation of disease burden and the impact of control interventions on this burden.
8. Research to increase the use and application of epidemiological models to aid M&E and surveillance, the design of cost-effective sampling protocols and the monitoring of intervention efficacy including drug resistance. These models should be linked to cost-effectiveness analyses of the interventions and their alternatives.

9. Research to investigate how helminth parasites modulate host–parasite interactions at the population and within-host levels, including the impact on the host immune response of concurrent infection with other helminth and non-helminth pathogens, the impact of parasite control interventions on such host–parasite interactions, and how concurrent infections affect clinical outcomes and the host's ability to seroconvert upon vaccination.
10. Research to annotate parasite genomes and transcriptomes, and to develop new tools for parasite functional genomics in key species.

Acknowledgements

The DRG4 especially wishes to acknowledge Dr Ayoade Oduola, Dr Johannes Sommerfeld, Dr Arve Lee Willingham, Dr Michael Wilson, Dr Deborah Kioy, Ms Edith Certain, Dr Julie Reza, Dr Margaret Harris and Ms Elisabetta Dessi from the Special Programme for Research and Training in Tropical Diseases (TDR), WHO, Geneva, Switzerland, who were instrumental in creating and managing the DRG, in preparing and coordinating the meetings, and in producing this report.

The DRG also acknowledges the advice and support of various groups and individuals from: WHO headquarters, Geneva, Switzerland, including Drs Lester Chitsulo, Dirk Engels and Dr Antonio Montresor of the Neglected Tropical Diseases (NTD) programme, and Dr Piero L. Olliaro of TDR; from the WHO Regional Office for Africa; from the WHO Country Office in Burkina Faso, including Drs Djamila Cabral, WHO Representative, and Guy-Michel Gershy-Damet, Regional Advisor for HIV Laboratory Programme, Focal Point HIV/ICST, and the WHO/Inter Country Support Team; and from the WHO Regional Office for the Americas (PAHO/AMRO).

Contributions made to the discussions during preparation of this report by the following stakeholders from the Ministry of Health, Burkina Faso are gratefully acknowledged: Dr Sylvestre Roger Marie Tiendrebeogo, Directeur, Direction de la Lutte contre la Maladie; Dr Sylvestre Tapsoba, Director of Nutrition; Dr Moussa Dadjoari, Coordinator for Schistosomiasis; Dr Emmanuel Seini, Neglected Tropical Diseases; and Mr Hamado Ouedraogo and Mr. Clément T. Bagnoa, both of the Schistosomiasis Control Programme. Also from Burkina Faso, the international and non-governmental organizations represented by: Dr Ann Tarini, Country Director, Helen Keller International; Mr Issouf Bamba, Project Coordinator, ONCHO-LF-VITAMIN A; Dr Seydou Toure, Country NTD Program Manager, RISEAL; Dr Maurice Hours, Chief of the Health and Nutrition Programme, United Nations Children's Fund (UNICEF); Dr Biram N'Diaye, nutrition specialist; and Dr Alhousseyni Maiga, FP/CPC. The group also recognized and acknowledged the valuable contributions from Prof Evariste Mutabatuka, Acting Director of the WHO/Multi Disease Surveillance Centre (MDSC), Burkina Faso, and from Dr Aimé Gilles Adjami, also of MDSC Burkina Faso.

Important contributions were made during the stakeholders' meeting in Rio de Janeiro, Brazil, by: Dr Zaida Yàdon, Regional Advisor on Communicable Diseases CDC/PAHO/AMRO, Rio de Janeiro, Brazil; Dr Ottorino Cosivi, Veterinary Public Health Unit Pan American Center for Foot and Mouth Disease (PANAFTOSA), Rio de Janeiro, Brazil; Dr Naftale Katz, Ministry of Health, Rio de Janeiro, Brazil; Dr Robert Bergquist, Ingerod, Sweden; Dr. Otavio Pieri, Oswaldo Cruz Foundation FIOCRUZ, Rio de Janeiro, Brazil; Dr Philip LoVerde, University of Texas Health Sciences Center, San Antonio, Texas, USA; Dr Jeffrey Bethony, George Washington University, USA; Professor P. Geldhof, Molecular Veterinary Parasitology, Department of Virology, Parasitology and Immunology, Faculty of Veterinary Medicine, Ghent University, Merelbeke, Belgium; and Professor Rodrigo Correa-Oliveira, Centro de Pesquisas Rene Rachou, FIOCRUZ MG, Belo Horizonte, Brazil.

The DRG4 also acknowledges the valuable support from the team at the African Programme for Onchocerciasis Control, Burkina Faso (where the first meeting of DRG4 was hosted), including from: Dr Uche Veronica Amazigo, Director; Dr Laurent Yameogo, Coordinator of the Director's Office; Dr Mounkaïla Noma, Chief of Epidemiology and Vector Elimination; Dr Grace Fobi, Community Ownership and Partnership Office; Dr Stephen Leak, Technical Adviser; Mrs. Zainab Akiwumi, Communication and Advocacy Officer; Mr. Paul Ejime, Communication Officer; Dr Afework Hailemariam Tekle, Epidemiologist; Mr. Saïdou N'Gadjaga, IT Help Desk Specialist; and Mr. Issaka Niadou Yacouba, Information System Officer.

Valuable advice and support was received from members of the Informal Consultation who helped identify the scope of DRG4, including: Professor Philip LoVerde, University of Texas Health Sciences Center, San Antonio, Texas, USA; Professor Roger Prichard, Institute of Parasitology, McGill University, Canada; Professor Rodrigo Correa-Oliveira, Centro de Pesquisas Rene Rachou, FIOCRUZ MG, Belo Horizonte, Brazil; Dr Warwick Grant, La Trobe University, Bundoora, Australia; Professor Xiao-Nong Zhou, Institute of Parasitic Diseases (IPD), Chinese Center for Diseases Control and Prevention (China CDC), Shanghai, People's Republic of China; Dr Daniel Boakye, Noguchi Memorial Institute of Medical Research, University of Ghana, Accra, Ghana; Professor Banchob Sripa, Khon Kaen University, Thailand.

The valuable contribution made in preparing this report by Dr. Mike Osei-Atweneboana, WHO/TDR Career Development fellow, from the Council for Scientific and Industrial Research, Ghana, is very much appreciated.

Finally, sincere thanks also to the peer reviewers for their comments and contributions to the technical accuracy of this report. Dr Nina Mattock was responsible for the technical editing.

TDR provided both technical and financial support for this report, and the European Commission provided financial support under Agreement PP-AP/2008/160-163.

References

1. Stoll NR. This wormy world. *Journal of Parasitology*, 1947, 33(1):1–18.
2. Hotez PJ et al. Control of neglected tropical diseases. *New England Journal of Medicine*, 2007, 357(10):1018–1027.
3. Hotez PJ et al. Helminth infections: the great neglected tropical diseases. *Journal of Clinical Investigation*, 2008, 118(4):1311–1321.
4. Hotez PJ et al. Rescuing the bottom billion through control of neglected tropical diseases. *Lancet*, 2009, 373(9674):1570–1575.
5. Zuehlke E. *Are parasitic worms a root cause of global poverty?* Population Reference Bureau, 2010 (http://prbblog.org/?p=137, accessed 28 February 2011).
6. *GSK increases support for WHO strategy to improve children's health with new 5-year commitment to expand donations of albendazole medicine: Increased donation to enable de-worming of all school age children in Africa*, GlaxoSmithKline media centre, 2010 (http://www.gsk.com/media/pressreleases/2010/2010_pressrelease_10110.htm, accessed 28 February 2011).
7. Brooker S et al. Contrasting patterns in the small-scale heterogeneity of human helminth infections in urban and rural environments in Brazil. *International Journal for Parasitology*, 2006, 36(10–11):1143–1151.
8. Kirby T, Molyneux D. Raising the profile of neglected tropical diseases. *Lancet*, 2010, 375(9708):21.
9. *Epidemiological profiles of neglected diseases and other infections related to poverty in Latin America and the Caribbean*. Washington DC, Pan American Health Organization, 2009 (http://new.paho.org/hq/index.php?option=com_content&task=view&id=1247&Itemid=211, accessed 28 February 2011).
10. Ault SK. Pan American Health Organization's Regional Strategic Framework for addressing neglected diseases in neglected populations in Latin America and the Caribbean. *Memórias do Instituto Oswaldo Cruz*, 2007, 102(Suppl 1):99–107.
11. Liese B, Rosenberg M, Schratz A. Programmes, partnerships, and governance for elimination and control of neglected tropical diseases. *Lancet*, 2010, 375(9708):67–76.
12. Remme JHF et al. Tropical diseases targeted for elimination: Chagas disease, lymphatic filariasis, onchocerciasis, and leprosy. In: Jamison DT, Breman JG and Measham AR, eds. *Disease control priorities in developing countries*, 2nd ed. New York, Oxford University Press, 2006:433–449.
13. Little MP et al. Association between microfilarial load and excess mortality in onchocerciasis: an epidemiological study. *Lancet*, 2004, 363(9420):1514–1521.
14. Basáñez MG et al. River blindness: a success story under threat? *PLoS Medicine*, 2006, 3(9):e371.
15. Murdoch ME. Onchodermatitis. *Current Opinion in Infectious Diseases*, 2010, 23(2):124–131.
16. *Strategic direction for research: lymphatic filariasis*. Geneva, Special Programme for Research and Training in Tropical Diseases, WHO, 2002 (http://www.who.int/tdr/diseases/lymphfil/direction.htm).
17. Ault SK. *Situación de las parasitosis desatendidas en América Latina y el Caribe y bases para un plan de acción para su eliminación*. OPS/OMS consensus meeting for an agenda on schistosomiasis research in the Americas, 2009 (Paraguay, October 22).
18. Guyatt HL, Bundy DAP. Estimating prevalence of community morbidity due to intestinal helminths: prevalence of infection as an indicator of the prevalence of disease. *Transactions of the Royal Society of Tropical Medicine and Hygiene*, 1991, 85(6):778–782.

19. de Silva NR, Chan MS, Bundy DAP. Morbidity and mortality due to ascariasis: re-estimation and sensitivity analysis of global numbers at risk. *Tropical Medicine & International Health*, 1997, 2(6):519–528.
20. de Silva NR, Guyatt HL, Bundy DAP. Morbidity and mortality due to Ascaris-induced intestinal obstruction. *Transactions of the Royal Society of Tropical Medicine and Hygiene*, 1997, 91(1):31–36.
21. Bundy DAP et al. The epidemiological implications of a multiple-infection approach to the control of human helminth infections. *Transactions of the Royal Society of Tropical Medicine and Hygiene*, 1991, 85(2):274–276.
22. Finkelstein JL et al. Decision-model estimation of the age-specific disability weight for schistosomiasis japonica: a systematic review of the literature. *PLoS Neglected Tropical Diseases*, 2008, 2(3):e158.
23. Steinmann P et al. Schistosomiasis and water resources development: systematic review, meta-analysis, and estimates of people at risk. *Lancet Infectious Diseases*, 2006, 6(7):411–425.
24. Chitsulo L et al. The global status of schistosomiasis and its control. *Acta Tropica*, 2000, 77(1):41–51.
25. Engels D et al. The global epidemiological situation of schistosomiasis and new approaches to control and research. *Acta Tropica*, 2002, 82(2):139–146.
26. van der Werf MJ et al. Quantification of clinical morbidity associated with schistosome infection in sub-Saharan Africa. *Acta Tropica*, 2003, 86(2–3):125–139.
27. King CH, Dickman K, Tisch DJ. Reassessment of the cost of chronic helmintic infection: a meta-analysis of disability-related outcomes in endemic schistosomiasis. *Lancet*, 2005, 365(9470):1561–1569.
28. Hotez PJ, Fenwick A. Schistosomiasis in Africa: an emerging tragedy in our new global health decade. *PLoS Neglected Tropical Diseases*, 2009, 3(9):e485.
29. Bergquist R, Johansen MV, Utzinger J. Diagnostic dilemmas in helminthology: what tools to use and when? *Trends in Parasitology*, 2009, 25(4):151–156.
30. Hatz C et al. Measurement of schistosomiasis-related morbidity at community level in areas of different endemicity. *Bulletin of the World Health Organization*, 1990, 68(6):777–787.
31. Webster JP et al. Evaluation and application of potential schistosome-associated morbidity markers within large-scale mass chemotherapy programmes. *Parasitology*, 2009, 136(13):1789–1799.
32. Wiest PM. The epidemiology of morbidity of schistosomiasis. *Parasitology Today*, 1996, 12(6):215–220.
33. Keiser J, Utzinger J. Food-borne trematodiases. *Clinical Microbiology Reviews*, 2009, 22(3):466–483.
34. Sanchez AL, Ljungstrom I, Medina MT. Diagnosis of human neurocysticercosis in endemic countries: a clinical study in Honduras. *Parasitology International*, 1999, 48(1):81–89.
35. Praet N et al. The disease burden of *Taenia solium* cysticercosis in Cameroon. *PLoS Neglected Tropical Diseases*, 2009, 3(3):e406.
36. Ndimubanzi PC et al. A systematic review of the frequency of neurocysticercosis with a focus on people with epilepsy. *PLoS Neglected Tropical Diseases*, 2010, 4(11):e870.
37. Brooker S et al. Epidemiology of single and multiple species of helminth infections among school children in Busia District, Kenya. *East African Medical Journal*, 2000, 77(3):157–161.
38. Faulkner H et al. Associations between filarial and gastrointestinal nematodes. *Transactions of the Royal Society of Tropical Medicine and Hygiene*, 2005, 99(4):301–312.
39. Canning D. Priority setting and the 'neglected' tropical diseases. *Transactions of the Royal Society of Tropical Medicine and Hygiene*, 2006, 100(6):499–504.

40. Hotez PJ et al. Incorporating a rapid-impact package for neglected tropical diseases with programs for HIV/AIDS, tuberculosis, and malaria. *PLoS Medicine*, 2006, 3(5):e102.
41. Chan M. *Address to the World Health Organization global partners meeting on neglected tropical diseases*. Geneva, World Health Organization, 2007 (http://www.who.int/dg/speeches/2007/190407_ntds/en/index.html, accessed 28 February 2012).
42. Mwangi TW, Bethony JM, Brooker S. Malaria and helminth interactions in humans: an epidemiological viewpoint. *Annals of Tropical Medicine and Parasitology*, 2006, 100(7):551–570.
43. Nacher M. Interactions between worm infections and malaria. *Clinical Reviews in Allergy and Immunology*, 2004, 26(2):85–92.
44. Supali T et al. Polyparasitism and its impact on the immune system. *International Journal for Parasitology*, 2010, 40(10):1171–1176.
45. WHO, *Global Health Observatory Map Gallery; topic: neglected tropical diseases*. Geneva, World Health Organization, 2011. (http://gamapserver.who.int/mapLibrary/, accessed 28 February 2011).
46. Colley DG, Secor WE. A schistosomiasis research agenda. *PLoS Neglected Tropical Diseases*, 2007, 1(3):e32.
47. Dujardin JC et al. Research priorities for neglected infectious diseases in Latin America and the Caribbean region. *PLoS Neglected Tropical Diseases*, 2010, 4(10):e780.
48. Foodborne trematode (FBT) infections and taeniasis/cysticercosis. In: *Report of a WHO Informal Consultation*. Vientiane, Lao People's Democratic Republic, 2009.
49. *Workshop on research priorities for neglected diseases in Brazil: schistosomiasis*. Brasilia, July 2008.
50. Guyatt HL et al. Evaluation of efficacy of school-based anthelmintic treatments against anaemia in children in the United Republic of Tanzania. *Bulletin of the World Health Organization*, 2001, 79(8):695–703.
51. Brooker S et al. Cost and cost-effectiveness of nationwide school-based helminth control in Uganda: intra-country variation and effects of scaling-up. *Health Policy and Planning*, 2008, 23(1):24–35.
52. Kabatereine NB et al. Impact of a national helminth control programme on infection and morbidity in Ugandan schoolchildren. *Bulletin of the World Health Organization*, 2007, 85(2):91–99.
53. Ramzy RM et al. Effect of yearly mass drug administration with diethylcarbamazine and albendazole on bancroftian filariasis in Egypt: a comprehensive assessment. *Lancet*, 2006, 367(9515):992–999.
54. Lindblade KA et al. Elimination of *Onchocerca volvulus* transmission in the Santa Rosa focus of Guatemala. *American Journal of Tropical Medicine and Hygiene*, 2007, 77(2):334–341.
55. Vieira JC et al. Impact of long-term treatment of onchocerciasis with ivermectin in Ecuador: potential for elimination of infection. *BMC Medicine*, 2007, 5:9.
56. Rodríguez-Pérez MA et al. Evidence for suppression of *Onchocerca volvulus* transmission in the Oaxaca focus in Mexico. *American Journal of Tropical Medicine and Hygiene*, 2008, 78(1):147–152.
57. Diawara L et al. Feasibility of onchocerciasis elimination with ivermectin treatment in endemic foci in Africa: first evidence from studies in Mali and Senegal. *PLoS Neglected Tropical Diseases*, 2009, 3(7):e497.
58. Little MP et al. Incidence of blindness during the Onchocerciasis Control Programme in western Africa, 1971–2002. *Journal of Infectious Diseases*, 2004, 189(10):1932–1941.
59. French MD et al. Observed reduction in *Schistosoma mansoni* transmission from large-scale administration of praziquantel in Uganda: A mathematical modelling study. *PLoS Neglected Tropical Diseases*, 2010, 4(11):e897.

60. Kolaczinski JH et al. Neglected tropical diseases in Uganda: the prospect and challenge of integrated control. *Trends in Parasitology*, 2007, 23(10):485–493.
61. Utzinger J et al. Schistosomiasis and neglected tropical diseases: towards integrated and sustainable control and a word of caution. *Parasitology*, 2009, 136(13):1859–1874.
62. Ramaiah KD et al. A programme to eliminate lymphatic filariasis in Tamil Nadu state, India: compliance with annual single-dose DEC mass treatment and some related operational aspects. *Tropical Medicine & International Health*, 2000, 5(12):842–847.
63. Ramaiah KD et al. Prolonged persistence of residual *Wuchereria bancrofti* infection after cessation of diethylcarbamazine-fortified salt programme. *Tropical Medicine & International Health*, 2009, 14(8):870–876.
64. Brady MA, Hooper PJ, Ottesen EA. Projected benefits from integrating NTD programs in sub-Saharan Africa. *Trends in Parasitology*, 2006, 22(7):285–291.
65. Brooker S, Utzinger J. Integrated disease mapping in a polyparasitic world. *Geospatial Health*, 2007, 1(2):141–146.
66. Bethony J et al. Soil-transmitted helminth infections: ascariasis, trichuriasis, and hookworm. *Lancet*, 2006, 367(9521):1521–1532.
67. Sousa-Figueiredo JC et al. Measuring morbidity associated with urinary schistosomiasis: assessing levels of excreted urine albumin and urinary tract pathologies. *PLoS Neglected Tropical Diseases*, 2009, 3(10):e526.
68. Vivas-Martinez S et al. Onchocerciasis in the Amazonian focus of southern Venezuela: altitude and blackfly species composition as predictors of endemicity to select communities for ivermectin control programmes. *Transactions of the Royal Society of Tropical Medicine and Hygiene*, 1998, 92(6):613–620.
69. Botto C et al. Geographical patterns of onchocerciasis in southern Venezuela: relationships between environment and infection prevalence. *Parassitologia*, 2005, 47(1):145–150.
70. Brooker S et al. An updated atlas of human helminth infections: the example of East Africa. *International Journal of Health Geographics*, 2009, 8:42.
71. Haas BJ et al. *Schistosoma mansoni* genome: closing in on a final gene set. *Experimental Parasitology*, 2007, 117(3):225–228.
72. Verjovski-Almeida S et al. Transcriptome analysis of the acoelomate human parasite *Schistosoma mansoni*. *Nature Genetics*, 2003, 35(2):148–157.
73. Liu F et al. New perspectives on host-parasite interplay by comparative transcriptomic and proteomic analyses of *Schistosoma japonicum*. *PLoS Pathogens*, 2006, 2(4):e29.
74. Ghedin E et al. Draft genome of the filarial nematode parasite *Brugia malayi*. *Science*, 2007, 317(5845):1756–1760.
75. Fitzpatrick JM et al. Anti-schistosomal intervention targets identified by lifecycle transcriptomic analyses. *PLoS Neglected Tropical Diseases*, 2009, 3(11):e543.
76. Gobert GN et al. Developmental gene expression profiles of the human pathogen *Schistosoma japonicum*. *BMC Genomics*, 2009,10:128.
77. Han ZG et al. *Schistosoma* genomics: new perspectives on schistosome biology and host-parasite interaction. *Annual Review of Genomics and Human Genetics*, 2009, 10:211–240.
78. Krautz-Peterson G et al. Optimizing gene suppression in schistosomes using RNA interference. *Molecular and Biochemical Parasitology*, 2007, 153(2):194–202.
79. Correnti JM, Brindley PJ, Pearce EJ. Long-term suppression of cathepsin B levels by RNA interference retards schistosome growth. *Molecular and Biochemical Parasitology*, 2005, 143(2):209–215.

80. Delcroix M et al. A multienzyme network functions in intestinal protein digestion by a platyhelminth parasite. *Journal of Biological Chemistry*, 2006, 281(51):39316–39329.
81. Freitas TC, Jung E, Pearce EJ. TGF-beta signaling controls embryo development in the parasitic flatworm *Schistosoma mansoni*. *PLoS Pathogens*, 2007, 3(4):e52.
82. Knox DP et al. RNA interference in parasitic nematodes of animals: a reality check? *Trends in Parasitology*, 2007, 23(3):105–107.
83. Viney ME, Thompson FJ. Two hypotheses to explain why RNA interference does not work in animal parasitic nematodes. *International Journal for Parasitology*, 2008, 38(1):43–47.
84. Maizels RM et al. Helminth parasites – masters of regulation. *Immunological Reviews*, 2004, 201:89–116.
85. Ohnmacht C, Voehringer D. Basophil effector function and homeostasis during helminth infection. *Blood*, 2009, 113(12):2816–2825.
86. Hartmann S, Lucius R. Modulation of host immune responses by nematode cystatins. *International Journal for Parasitology*, 2003, 33(11):1291–1302.
87. Harnett W, McInnes IB, Harnett MM. ES-62, a filarial nematode-derived immunomodulator with anti-inflammatory potential. *Immunology Letters*, 2004, 94(1-2):27–33.
88. Lima C et al. Eosinophilic inflammation and airway hyper-responsiveness are profoundly inhibited by a helminth (*Ascaris suum*) extract in a murine model of asthma. *Clinical and Experimental Allergy*, 2002, 32(11):1659–1666.
89. Schnoeller C et al. A helminth immunomodulator reduces allergic and inflammatory responses by induction of IL-10-producing macrophages. *Journal of Immunology*, 2008, 180(6):4265–4272.
90. Berriman M et al. The genome of the blood fluke *Schistosoma mansoni*. *Nature*, 2009, 460(7253):352–358.
91. Brattig NW. Pathogenesis and host responses in human onchocerciasis: impact of *Onchocerca filariae* and *Wolbachia* endobacteria. *Microbes and Infection*, 2004, 6(1):113–128.
92. Pastrana DV et al. Filarial nematode parasites secrete a homologue of the human cytokine macrophage migration inhibitory factor. *Infection and Immunity*, 1998, 66(12):5955–5963.
93. Foster J et al. The *Wolbachia* genome of *Brugia malayi*: endosymbiont evolution within a human pathogenic nematode. *PLoS Biology*, 2005, 3(4):e121.
94. Taylor MJ, Hoerauf A, Bockarie M. Lymphatic filariasis and onchocerciasis. *Lancet*, 2010, 376(9747):1175–1185.
95. Penzer R. Lymphatic filariasis and the role of nursing interventions. *Journal of Lymphoedema*, 2007, 2:48–53.
96. Boussinesq M et al. Clinical picture, epidemiology and outcome of *Loa*-associated serious adverse events related to mass ivermectin treatment of onchocerciasis in Cameroon. *Filaria Journal*, 2003, 2(Suppl 1):S4.
97. Basáñez MG et al. Effect of single-dose ivermectin on *Onchocerca volvulus*: a systematic review and meta-analysis. *Lancet Infectious Diseases*, 2008, 8(5):310–322.
98. Michael E et al. Mathematical modelling and the control of lymphatic filariasis. *Lancet Infectious Diseases*, 2004, 4(4):223–234.
99. Tisch DJ, Michael E, Kazura JW. Mass chemotherapy options to control lymphatic filariasis: a systematic review. *Lancet Infectious Diseases*, 2005, 5(8):514–523.
100. Diawara A. *Development of DNA assays for the detection of single nucleotide polymorphism associated with benzimidazole resistance, in human soil-transmitted helminths*. Thesis, McGill University Institute of Parasitology, Montreal. Canada, McGill University, 2008.

101. Sabah AA et al. *Schistosoma mansoni*: chemotherapy of infections of different ages. *Experimental Parasitology*, 1986, 61(3):294–303.
102. Utzinger J et al. Artemisinins for schistosomiasis and beyond. *Current Opinion in Investigational Drugs*, 2007, 8(2):105–116.
103. Huyse T et al. Bidirectional introgressive hybridization between a cattle and human schistosome species. *PLoS Pathogens*, 2009, 5(9):e1000571.
104. Rudge JW et al. Parasite genetic differentiation by habitat type and host species: molecular epidemiology of *Schistosoma japonicum* in hilly and marshland areas of Anhui Province, China. *Molecular Ecology*, 2009, 18(10):2134–2147.
105. Lu DB et al. Contrasting reservoirs for *Schistosoma japonicum* between marshland and hilly regions in Anhui, China – a two-year longitudinal parasitological survey. *Parasitology*, 2010, 137(1):99–110.
106. Rudge JW et al. Population genetics of *Schistosoma japonicum* within the Philippines suggest high levels of transmission between humans and dogs. *PLoS Neglected Tropical Diseases*, 2008, 2(11):e340.
107. Riley S et al. Multi-host transmission dynamics of *Schistosoma japonicum* in Samar province, the Philippines. *PLoS Medicine*, 2008, 5(1):e18.
108. Wu HW et al. High prevalence of *Schistosoma japonicum* infection in water buffaloes in the Philippines assessed by real-time polymerase chain reaction. *American Journal of Tropical Medicine and Hygiene*, 2010, 82(4):646–652.
109. Garba A et al. Present and future schistosomiasis control activities with support from the Schistosomiasis Control Initiative in West Africa. *Parasitology*, 2009, 136(13):1731–1737.
110. Touré S et al. Two-year impact of single praziquantel treatment on infection in the national control programme on schistosomiasis in Burkina Faso. *Bulletin of the World Health Organization*, 2008, 86(10):780–787.
111. Zhang Y et al. Parasitological impact of 2-year preventive chemotherapy on schistosomiasis and soil-transmitted helminthiasis in Uganda. *BMC Medicine*, 2007, 5:27.
112. Clements AC et al. Use of Bayesian geostatistical prediction to estimate local variations in *Schistosoma haematobium* infection in western Africa. *Bulletin of the World Health Organization*, 2009, 87(12):921–929.
113. Clements AC et al. Spatial co-distribution of neglected tropical diseases in the east African great lakes region: revisiting the justification for integrated control. *Tropical Medicine & International Health*, 2010, 15(2):198–207.
114. Brooker S et al. Rapid assessment of *Schistosoma mansoni*: the validity, applicability and cost-effectiveness of the Lot Quality Assurance Sampling method in Uganda. *Tropical Medicine & International Health*, 2005, 10(7):647–658.
115. Sripa B et al. Liver fluke induces cholangiocarcinoma. *PLoS Medicine*, 2007, 4(7):e201.
116. Garcia HH et al. Strategies for the elimination of taeniasis/cysticercosis. *Journal of Neurological Sciences*, 2007, 262(1-2):153–157.
117. Lightowlers MW. Eradication of *Taenia solium* cysticercosis: A role for vaccination of pigs. *International Journal for Parasitology*, 2010, 40(10):1183–1192.
118. Assana E et al. Elimination of *Taenia solium* transmission to pigs in a field trial of the TSOL18 vaccine in Cameroon. *International Journal for Parasitology*, 2010, 40(5):515–519.
119. French MD et al. School-based control of urinary schistosomiasis on Zanzibar, Tanzania: monitoring micro-haematuria with reagent strips as a rapid urological assessment. *Journal of Pediatric Urology*, 2007, 3(5):364–368.

120. Massa K et al. Community perceptions on the community-directed treatment and school-based approaches for the control of schistosomiasis and soil-transmitted helminthiasis among school-age children in Lushoto District, Tanzania. *Journal of Biosocial Science*, 2009, 41(1):89–105.

121. Massa K et al. The effect of the community-directed treatment approach versus the school-based treatment approach on the prevalence and intensity of schistosomiasis and soil-transmitted helminthiasis among schoolchildren in Tanzania. *Transactions of the Royal Society of Tropical Medicine and Hygiene*, 2009, 103(1):31–37.

122. Brooker S, Clements AC, Bundy DAP. Global epidemiology, ecology and control of soil-transmitted helminth infections. *Advances in Parasitology*, 2006, 62:221–261.

123. Mohammed KA et al. Triple co-administration of ivermectin, albendazole and praziquantel in Zanzibar: a safety study. *PLoS Neglected Tropical Diseases*, 2008, 2(1):e171.

124. Olsen A. Efficacy and safety of drug combinations in the treatment of schistosomiasis, soil-transmitted helminthiasis, lymphatic filariasis and onchocerciasis. *Transactions of the Royal Society of Tropical Medicine and Hygiene*, 2007,101(8):747–758.

125. Bundy DA et al. Deworming and development: asking the right questions, asking the questions right. *PLoS Neglected Tropical Diseases*, 2009, 3(1):e362.

126. Smits HL. Prospects for the control of neglected tropical diseases by mass drug administration. *Expert Review of Anti-infective Therapy*, 2009, 7(1):37–56.

127. Churcher TS et al. Identifying sub-optimal responses to ivermectin in the treatment of river blindness. *Proceedings of the National Academy of Sciences of the United States of America*, 2009, 106(39):16716–16721.

128. Churcher TS, Basáñez MG. Sampling strategies to detect anthelmintic resistance: the perspective of human onchocerciasis. *Trends in Parasitology*, 2009, 25(1):11–17.

129. Mathieu E et al. Comparison of methods for estimating drug coverage for filariasis elimination, Leogane Commune, Haiti. *Transactions of the Royal Society of Tropical Medicine and Hygiene*, 2003, 97(5):501–505.

130. Geary TG et al. Unresolved issues in anthelmintic pharmacology for helminthiases of humans. *International Journal for Parasitology*, 2010, 40(1):1–13.

131. Ramaiah KD. Lymphatic filariasis elimination programme in India: progress and challenges. *Trends in Parasitology*, 2009, 25(1):7–8.

132. Wanji S et al. Community-directed delivery of doxycycline for the treatment of onchocerciasis in areas of co-endemicity with loiasis in Cameroon. *Parasites & Vectors*, 2009, 2(1):39.

133. Bourguinat C et al., (2010) Analysis of the mdr-1 gene in patients co-infected with *Onchocerca volvulus* and *Loa loa* who experienced a post-ivermectin serious adverse event. *American Journal of Tropical Medicine and Hygiene* 83(1):28–32.

134. Diawara A et al. Assays to detect beta-tubulin codon 200 polymorphism in *Trichuris trichiura* and *Ascaris lumbricoides*. *PLoS Neglected Tropical Diseases*, 2009, 3(3):e397.

135. McManus DP, Loukas A. Current status of vaccines for schistosomiasis. *Clinical Microbiology Reviews*, 2008, 21(1):225–242.

136. Doenhoff MJ et al. Chemotherapy and drug resistance in schistosomiasis, fascioliasis and tapeworm infections. In: Mayers DL ed. *Antimicrobial Drug Resistance, Volume 1, mechanisms of drug resistance*. London, Humana Press, 2009:629–646.

137. Lightowlers MW. Vaccination for the prevention of cysticercosis. *Developments in Biologicals (Basel)*, 2004, 119:361–368.

138. Keiser J, Utzinger J. Efficacy of current drugs against soil-transmitted helminth infections: systematic review and meta-analysis. *Journal of the American Medical Association*, 2008, 299(16):1937–1948.

139. Stepek G et al. Human gastrointestinal nematode infections: are new control methods required? *International Journal of Experimental Pathology*, 2006, 87(5):325–341.

140. Hu Y, Xiao SH, Aroian RV. The new anthelmintic tribendimidine is an L-type (levamisole and pyrantel) nicotinic acetylcholine receptor agonist. *PLoS Neglected Tropical Diseases*, 2009, 3(8):e499.

141. Wolstenholme AJ et al. Drug resistance in veterinary helminths. *Trends in Parasitology*, 2004, 20(10):469–476.

142. Martin PJ, Anderson N, Jarrett RG. Detecting benzimidazole resistance with faecal egg count reduction tests and in vitro assays. *Australian Veterinary Journal*, 1989, 66(8):236–240.

143. De Clercq D et al. Failure of mebendazole in treatment of human hookworm infections in the southern region of Mali. *American Journal of Tropical Medicine and Hygiene*, 1997, 57(1):25–30.

144. Sacko M et al. Comparison of the efficacy of mebendazole, albendazole and pyrantel in treatment of human hookworm infections in the southern region of Mali, West Africa. *Transactions of the Royal Society of Tropical Medicine and Hygiene*, 1999, 93(2):195–203.

145. Reynoldson JA et al. Failure of pyrantel in treatment of human hookworm infections (*Ancylostoma duodenale*) in the Kimberley region of north west Australia. *Acta Tropica*, 1997, 68(3):301–312.

146. Albonico M et al. Efficacy of mebendazole and levamisole alone or in combination against intestinal nematode infections after repeated targeted mebendazole treatment in Zanzibar. *Bulletin of the World Health Organization*, 2003, 81(5):343–352.

147. Flohr C et al. Low efficacy of mebendazole against hookworm in Vietnam: two randomized controlled trials. *American Journal of Tropical Medicine and Hygiene*, 2007, 76(4):732–736.

148. Albonico M, Wright V, Bickle Q. Molecular analysis of the beta-tubulin gene of human hookworms as a basis for possible benzimidazole resistance on Pemba Island. *Molecular and Biochemical Parasitology*, 2004, 134(2):281–284.

149. Schwenkenbecher JM et al. Characterization of beta-tubulin genes in hookworms and investigation of resistance-associated mutations using real-time PCR. *Molecular and Biochemical Parasitology*, 2007, 156(2):167–174.

150. Eberhard ML, Lowrie RC Jr., Lammie PJ. Persistence of microfilaremia in bancroftian filariasis after diethylcarbamazine citrate therapy. *Tropical Medicine and Parasitology*, 1988, 39(2):128–130.

151. Eberhard ML et al. Evidence of nonsusceptibility to diethylcarbamazine in *Wuchereria bancrofti*. *Journal of Infectious Diseases*, 1991, 163(5):1157–1160.

152. Dixit V, Gupta AK, Prasad GB. Interruption of annual single dose DEC regimen administration: impact on *Wuchereria bancrofti* microfilaraemia, vector infection and infectivity rates. *Journal of Communicable Diseases*, 2009, 41(1):25–31.

153. Schwab AE et al. Detection of benzimidazole resistance-associated mutations in the filarial nematode Wuchereria bancrofti and evidence for selection by albendazole and ivermectin combination treatment. *American Journal of Tropical Medicine and Hygiene*, 2005, 73(2):234–238.

154. Bourguinat C et al. Genetic selection of low fertile *Onchocerca volvulus* by ivermectin treatment. *PLoS Neglected Tropical Diseases*, 2007, 1(1):e72.

155. Eng JK, Prichard RK. A comparison of genetic polymorphism in populations of *Onchocerca volvulus* from untreated- and ivermectin-treated patients. *Molecular and Biochemical Parasitology*, 2005, 142(2):193–202.

156. Eng JK et al. Ivermectin selection on beta-tubulin: evidence in *Onchocerca volvulus* and *Haemonchus contortus*. *Molecular and Biochemical Parasitology*, 2006, 150(2):229–235.

157. Awadzi K et al. An investigation of persistent microfilaridermias despite multiple treatments with ivermectin, in two onchocerciasis-endemic foci in Ghana. *Annals of Tropical Medicine and Parasitology*, 2004, 98(3):231–249.

158. Awadzi K et al. Thirty-month follow-up of sub-optimal responders to multiple treatments with ivermectin, in two onchocerciasis-endemic foci in Ghana. *Annals of Tropical Medicine and Parasitology*, 2004, 98(4):359–370.

159. Osei-Atweneboana MY et al. Prevalence and intensity of *Onchocerca volvulus* infection and efficacy of ivermectin in endemic communities in Ghana: a two-phase epidemiological study. *Lancet*, 2007, 369(9578):2021–2029.

160. Bourguinat C et al. P-glycoprotein-like protein, a possible genetic marker for ivermectin resistance selection in *Onchocerca volvulus*. *Molecular and Biochemical Parasitology*, 2008, 158(2):101–111.

161. Ardelli BF, Prichard RK. Identification of variant ABC-transporter genes among *Onchocerca volvulus* collected from ivermectin-treated and untreated patients in Ghana, West Africa. *Annals of Tropical Medicine and Parasitology*, 2004, 98(4):371–384.

162. Ardelli BF, Guerriero SB, Prichard RK. Genomic organization and effects of ivermectin selection on *Onchocerca volvulus* P-glycoprotein. *Molecular and Biochemical Parasitology*, 2005, 143(1):58–66.

163. Ardelli BF, Prichard RK. Reduced genetic variation of an *Onchocerca volvulus* ABC transporter gene following treatment with ivermectin. *Transactions of the Royal Society of Tropical Medicine and Hygiene*, 2007, 101(12):1223–1232.

164. Ardelli BF, Guerriero SB, Prichard RK. Characterization of a half-size ATP-binding cassette transporter gene which may be a useful marker for ivermectin selection in *Onchocerca volvulus*. *Molecular and Biochemical Parasitology*, 2006, 145(1):94–100.

165. Ardelli BF, Guerriero SB, Prichard RK. Ivermectin imposes selection pressure on P-glycoprotein from *Onchocerca volvulus*: linkage disequilibrium and genotype diversity. *Parasitology*, 2006, 132(3):375–386.

166. Remme JH et al. Efficacy of ivermectin against *Onchocerca volvulus* in Ghana. *Lancet*, 2007, 370(9593):1123–1124.

167. Dobson RJ et al. Principles for the use of macrocyclic lactones to minimise selection for resistance. *Australian Veterinary Journal*, 2001, 79(11):756–761.

168. Leathwick DM et al. Managing anthelmintic resistance: is it feasible in New Zealand to delay the emergence of resistance to a new anthelmintic class? *New Zealand Veterinary Journal*, 2009, 57(4):181–192.

169. Coles GC, Roush RT. Slowing the spread of anthelmintic resistant nematodes of sheep and goats in the United Kingdom. *Veterinary Record*, 1992, 130(23):505–510.

170. van Wyk JA. Refugia – overlooked as perhaps the most potent factor concerning the development of anthelmintic resistance. *Onderstepoort Journal of Veterinary Research*, 2001, 68(1):55–67.

171. Wood RJ, Mani GS. The effective dominance of resistance genes in relation to the evolution of resistance. *Pesticide Science*, 1981, 12:573–581.

172. Curtis CF. Theoretical models of the use of insecticide mixtures for the management of resistance. *Bulletin of Entomological Research*, 1985, 75:259–265.

173. Mani GS. Evolution of resistance in the presence of two insecticides. *Genetics*, 1985, 109:761–783.

174. Comins HN. Tactics for resistance management using multiple pesticides. *Agriculture, Ecosystems and Environment*, 1986, 16:129–148.
175. Roush RT. Designing resistance management programs: how can you choose? *Pesticide Science*, 1989, 26:423–441.
176. Tabashnik BE. Managing resistance with multiple pesticide tactics: theory, evidence, and recommendations. *Journal of Economic Entomology*, 1989, 82:1263–1269.
177. Prichard RK. Ivermectin resistance and overview of the Consortium for Anthelmintic Resistance SNPs. *Expert Opinion on Drug Discovery*, 2007, 2(Suppl.1):S41–S52.
178. Lespine A et al. ABC transporter modulation: a strategy to enhance the activity of macrocyclic lactone anthelmintics. *Trends in Parasitology*, 2008, 24(7):293–298.
179. Kerboeuf D et al. P-glycoprotein in helminths: function and perspectives for anthelmintic treatment and reversal of resistance. *International Journal of Antimicrobial Agents*, 2003, 22(3):332–346.
180. Blackhall WJ, Prichard RK, Beech RN. P-glycoprotein selection in strains of *Haemonchus contortus* resistant to benzimidazoles. *Veterinary Parasitology*, 2008, 152(1-2):101–107.
181. von Samson-Himmelstjerna G, Prichard RK, Wolstenholme AJ. Anthelmintic resistance as a guide to the discovery of new drugs. In: Selzer P, ed. *Drug discovery in infectious diseases*. Weinheim, Wiley-VCH, 2009:17–32.
182. de Lourdes Mottier M, Prichard RK. Genetic analysis of a relationship between macrocyclic lactone and benzimidazole anthelmintic selection on *Haemonchus contortus*. *Pharmacogenetics and Genomics*, 2008, 18(2):129–140.
183. Williamson SA et al. Investigating candidate resistance genes in an ivermectin-resistant isolate of *Haemonchus contortus*. In: *American Association of Veterinary Parasitologists 55th Annual Meeting*. Atlanta, GA, USA, 2010.
184. Awadzi K et al. The safety, tolerability and pharmacokinetics of levamisole alone, levamisole plus ivermectin, and levamisole plus albendazole, and their efficacy against *Onchocerca volvulus*. *Annals of Tropical Medicine and Parasitology*, 2004, 98(6):595–614.
185. Hougard JM et al. Eliminating onchocerciasis after 14 years of vector control: a proved strategy. *Journal of Infectious Diseases*, 2001, 184(4):497–503.
186. Utzinger J et al. Conquering schistosomiasis in China: the long march. *Acta Tropica*, 2005, 96(2-3):69–96.
187. Curtis CF et al. Use of floating layers of polystyrene beads to control populations of the filaria vector *Culex quinquefasciatus*. *Annals of Tropical Medicine and Parasitology*, 2002, 96(Suppl 2):S97–104.
188. Sunish IP et al. Vector control complements mass drug administration against bancroftian filariasis in Tirukoilur, India. *Bulletin of the World Health Organization*, 2007, 85(2):138–145.
189. Davies JB. Sixty years of onchocerciasis vector control: a chronological summary with comments on eradication, reinvasion, and insecticide resistance. *Annual Review of Entomology*, 1994, 39:23–45.
190. Hotez PJ, Ferris MT. The antipoverty vaccines. *Vaccine*, 2006, 24(31–32):5787–5799.
191. Hotez PJ, Brown AS. Neglected tropical disease vaccines. *Biologicals*, 2009, 37(3):160–164.
192. Ghosh K et al. The impact of concurrent and treated *Ancylostoma ceylanicum* hookworm infections on the immunogenicity of a recombinant hookworm vaccine in hamsters. *Journal of Infectious Diseases*, 2006, 193(1):155–162.
193. Mutapi F et al. Praziquantel treatment of individuals exposed to *Schistosoma haematobium* enhances serological recognition of defined parasite antigens. *Journal of Infectious Diseases*, 2005, 192(6):1108–1118.

194. Hotez PJ et al. Multivalent anthelminthic vaccine to prevent hookworm and schistosomiasis. *Expert Review of Vaccines*, 2008, 7(6):745–752.

195. Lustigman S, Abraham D. Onchocerciasis. In: Barrett ADT, Stanberry LR, eds. *Vaccines for biodefense and emerging and neglected diseases*. Academic Press Inc - Elsevier Science & Technology, 2009, chapter 67:1379–1400.

196. Hotez PJ et al. Vaccines for hookworm infection. *Pediatric Infectious Disease Journal*, 1997, 16(10):935–940.

197. Bergquist R, Lustigman S. Control of important helminthic infections: vaccine development as part of the solution. *Advances in Parasitology*, 2010, 73:297–326.

198. Ngoumou P, Walsh JF, Mace JM. A rapid mapping technique for the prevalence and distribution of onchocerciasis: a Cameroon case study. *Annals of Tropical Medicine and Parasitology*, 1994, 88(5):463–474.

199. Lengeler C et al. Community-based questionnaires and health statistics as tools for the cost-efficient identification of communities at risk of urinary schistosomiasis. *International Journal of Epidemiology*, 1991, 20(3):796–807.

200. Wanji S et al. Combined utilisation of rapid assessment procedures for loiasis (RAPLOA) and onchocerciasis (REA) in rain forest villages of Cameroon. *Filaria Journal*, 2005, 4(1):2.

201. Boatin BA, Richards FO Jr. Control of onchocerciasis. *Advances in Parasitology*, 2006, 61:349–394.

202. Boatin BA et al. Detection of *Onchocerca volvulus* infection in low prevalence areas: a comparison of three diagnostic methods. *Parasitology*, 2002, 125(6):545–552.

203. Chambers EW et al. Xenomonitoring of *Wuchereria bancrofti* and *Dirofilaria immitis* infections in mosquitoes from American Samoa: trapping considerations and a comparison of polymerase chain reaction assays with dissection. *American Journal of Tropical Medicine and Hygiene*, 2009, 80(5):774–781.

204. Lipner EM et al. Field applicability of a rapid-format anti-Ov-16 antibody test for the assessment of onchocerciasis control measures in regions of endemicity. *Journal of Infectious Diseases*, 2006, 194(2):216–221.

205. Lammie PJ et al. Recombinant antigen-based antibody assays for the diagnosis and surveillance of lymphatic filariasis – a multicenter trial. *Filaria Journal*, 2004, 3(1):9.

206. Mladonicky JM et al. Assessing transmission of lymphatic filariasis using parasitologic, serologic, and entomologic tools after mass drug administration in American Samoa. *American Journal of Tropical Medicine and Hygiene*, 2009, 80(5):769–773.

207. Cringoli G. FLOTAC, a novel apparatus for a multivalent faecal egg count technique. *Parassitologia*, 2006, 48(3):381–384.

208. World Health Organization. *Elimination of schistosomiasis from low-transmission areas: Report of a WHO Informal Consultation 18–19 August 2008*. Salvador, Bahia, Brazil, 2009.

209. Zhu YC. Immunodiagnosis and its role in schistosomiasis control in China: a review. *Acta Tropica*, 2005, 96(2–3):130–136.

210. Lier T et al. Real-time polymerase chain reaction for detection of low-intensity *Schistosoma japonicum* infections in China. *American Journal of Tropical Medicine and Hygiene*, 2009, 81(3):428–432.

211. Handali S et al. Development and evaluation of a magnetic immunochromatographic test to detect *Taenia solium*, which causes taeniasis and neurocysticercosis in humans. *Clinical and Vaccine Immunology*, 2010, 17(4):631–637.

212. Guezala MC et al. Development of a species-specific coproantigen ELISA for human *Taenia solium* taeniasis. *American Journal of Tropical Medicine and Hygiene*, 2009, 81(3):433–437.
213. Taylor HR et al. Sensitivity of skin snips in the diagnosis of onchocerciasis. *Tropical Medicine and Parasitology*, 1987, 38(2):145–147.
214. Stingl P et al. A diagnostic "patch test" for onchocerciasis using topical diethylcarbamazine. *Transactions of the Royal Society of Tropical Medicine and Hygiene*, 1984, 78(2):254–258.
215. Lindblade KA et al. Elimination of *Onchocerca volvulus* transmission in the Santa Rosa focus of Guatemala. *American Journal of Tropical Medicine and Hygiene*, 2007, 77(2):334–341.
216. Rodríguez-Pérez MA et al. Antibody detection tests for Onchocerca volvulus: comparison of the sensitivity of a cocktail of recombinant antigens used in the indirect enzyme-linked immunosorbent assay with a rapid-format antibody card test. *Transactions of the Royal Society of Tropical Medicine and Hygiene*, 2003, 97(5):539–541.
217. Burbelo PD et al. A four-antigen mixture for rapid assessment of *Onchocerca volvulus* infection. *PLoS Neglected Tropical Diseases*, 2009, 3(5):e438.
218. Klion AD et al. Serum immunoglobulin G4 antibodies to the recombinant antigen, LI-SXP-1, are highly specific for *Loa loa* infection. *Journal of Infectious Diseases*, 2003, 187(1):128–133.
219. Rahmah N et al. A recombinant antigen-based IgG4 ELISA for the specific and sensitive detection of Brugia malayi infection. *Transactions of the Royal Society of Tropical Medicine and Hygiene*, 2001, 95(3):280–284.
220. More SJ, Copeman DB. A highly specific and sensitive monoclonal antibody-based ELISA for the detection of circulating antigen in bancroftian filariasis. *Tropical Medicine and Parasitology*, 1990, 41(4):403–406.
221. Weil GJ et al. A monoclonal antibody-based enzyme immunoassay for detecting parasite antigenemia in bancroftian filariasis. *Journal of Infectious Diseases*, 1987, 156(2):350–355.
222. McCarthy JS et al. Clearance of circulating filarial antigen as a measure of the macrofilaricidal activity of diethylcarbamazine in *Wuchereria bancrofti* infection. *Journal of Infectious Diseases*, 1995, 172(2):521–526.
223. Onapa AW et al. Rapid assessment of the geographical distribution of lymphatic filariasis in Uganda, by screening of schoolchildren for circulating filarial antigens. *Annals of Tropical Medicine and Parasitology*, 2005, 99(2):141–153.
224. Toé L et al. Detection of *Onchocerca volvulus* infection by O-150 polymerase chain reaction analysis of skin scratches. *Journal of Infectious Diseases*, 1998, 178(1):282–285.
225. Zhong M et al. A polymerase chain reaction assay for detection of the parasite *Wuchereria bancrofti* in human blood samples. *American Journal of Tropical Medicine and Hygiene*, 1996, 54(4):357–363.
226. Basáñez MG et al. Determination of sample sizes for the estimation of *Onchocerca volvulus* (Filarioidea: Onchocercidae) infection rates in biting populations of *Simulium ochraceum* s.l. (Diptera: Simuliidae) and its application to ivermectin control programs. *Journal of Medical Entomology*, 1998, 35(5):745–757.
227. Duerr HP, Raddatz G, Eichner M. Diagnostic value of nodule palpation in onchocerciasis. *Transactions of the Royal Society of Tropical Medicine and Hygiene*, 2008, 102(2):148–154.
228. Mand S et al. Frequent detection of worm movements in onchocercal nodules by ultrasonography. *Filaria Journal*, 2005, 4(1):1.
229. Dreyer G et al. Direct assessment of the adulticidal efficacy of a single dose of ivermectin in bancroftian filariasis. *Transactions of the Royal Society of Tropical Medicine and Hygiene*, 1995, 89(4):441–443.

230. Ozoh G et al. Evaluation of the diethylcarbamazine patch to evaluate onchocerciasis endemicity in Central Africa. *Tropical Medicine & International Health*, 2007, 12(1):123–129.
231. Gyapong JO et al. The use of spatial analysis in mapping the distribution of bancroftian filariasis in four West African countries. *Annals of Tropical Medicine and Parasitology*, 2002, 96(7):695–705.
232. Gardon J et al. Serious reactions after mass treatment of onchocerciasis with ivermectin in an area endemic for *Loa loa* infection. *Lancet*, 1997, 350(9070):18-22.
233. Diggle P, Tawn J, Moyeed R. Model-based geostatistics. *Journal of the Royal Statistical Society*, Series C (Applied Statistics), 1998, 47(3):299–350.
234. Thomson MC et al. Satellite mapping of *Loa loa* prevalence in relation to ivermectin use in west and central Africa. *Lancet*, 2000, 356(9235):1077–1078.
235. Takougang I et al. Rapid assessment method for prevalence and intensity of *Loa loa* infection. *Bulletin of the World Health Organization*, 2002, 80(11):852–858.
236. Crainiceanu C, Diggle P, Rowlingson B. Bivariate binomial spatial modeling of *Loa loa* prevalence in tropical Africa. *Journal of the American Statistical Association*, 2008, 103(481):21–38.
237. Gonzalez RJ et al. Successful interruption of transmission of *Onchocerca volvulus* in the Escuintla-Guatemala focus, Guatemala. *PLoS Neglected Tropical Diseases*, 2009, 3(3):e404.
238. Basáñez MG, Churcher TS, Grillet ME. *Onchocerca-Simulium* interactions and the population and evolutionary biology of *Onchocerca volvulus*. *Advances in Parasitology*, 2009, 68:263–313.
239. Gambhir M, Michael E. Complex ecological dynamics and eradicability of the vector borne macroparasitic disease, lymphatic filariasis. *PLoS ONE* 2008, 3(8):e2874.
240. Churcher TS, Basáñez MG. Density dependence and the spread of anthelmintic resistance. *Evolution*, 2008, 62(3):528–537.
241. Churcher TS et al. An analysis of genetic diversity and inbreeding in *Wuchereria bancrofti*: implications for the spread and detection of drug resistance. *PLoS Neglected Tropical Diseases*, 2008, 2(4):e211.
242. Schwab AE et al. An analysis of the population genetics of potential multi-drug resistance in *Wuchereria bancrofti* due to combination chemotherapy. *Parasitology*, 2007, 134(7):1025–1040.
243. Schwab AE et al. Population genetics of concurrent selection with albendazole and ivermectin or diethylcarbamazine on the possible spread of albendazole resistance in *Wuchereria bancrofti*. *Parasitology*, 2006, 133(5):589–601.
244. Walker M et al. Density-dependent effects on the weight of female *Ascaris lumbricoides* infections of humans and its impact on patterns of egg production. *Parasites & Vectors*, 2009, 2(1):11.
245. Bungiro RD Jr., Cappello M. Detection of excretory/secretory coproantigens in experimental hookworm infection. *American Journal of Tropical Medicine and Hygiene*, 2005, 73(5):915–920.
246. Verweij JJ et al. Simultaneous detection and quantification of *Ancylostoma duodenale*, *Necator americanus*, and *Oesophagostomum bifurcum* in fecal samples using multiplex real-time PCR. *American Journal of Tropical Medicine and Hygiene*, 2007, 77(4):685–690.
247. de Gruijter JM et al. Polymerase chain reaction-based differential diagnosis of *Ancylostoma duodenale* and *Necator americanus* infections in humans in northern Ghana. *Tropical Medicine & International Health*, 2005, 10(6):574–580.
248. Goodman D et al. A comparison of methods for detecting the eggs of *Ascaris*, *Trichuris*, and hookworm in infant stool, and the epidemiology of infection in Zanzibari infants. *American Journal of Tropical Medicine and Hygiene*, 2007, 76(4):725–731.
249. Rossanigo CE, Gruner L. Accuracy of two methods for counting eggs of sheep nematode parasites. *Veterinary Parasitology*, 1991, 39(1-2):115–121.

250. Knopp S et al. A single FLOTAC is more sensitive than triplicate Kato-Katz for the diagnosis of low-intensity soil-transmitted helminth infections. *Transactions of the Royal Society of Tropical Medicine and Hygiene*, 2009, 103(4):347–354.

251. Utzinger J et al. FLOTAC: a new sensitive technique for the diagnosis of hookworm infections in humans. *Transactions of the Royal Society of Tropical Medicine and Hygiene*, 2008, 102(1):84–90.

252. Bennett A, Guyatt H. Reducing intestinal nematode infection: efficacy of albendazole and mebendazole. *Parasitology Today*, 2000, 16(2):71–74.

253. Coles GC et al. The detection of anthelmintic resistance in nematodes of veterinary importance. *Veterinary Parasitology*, 2006, 136(3-4):167–185.

254. Kotze AC, Kopp SR. The potential impact of density dependent fecundity on the use of the faecal egg count reduction test for detecting drug resistance in human hookworms. *PLoS Neglected Tropical Diseases*, 2008, 2(10):e297.

255. Hall A, Holland C. Geographical variation in *Ascaris lumbricoides* fecundity and its implications for helminth control. *Parasitology Today*, 2000, 16(12):540–544.

256. Kotze AC et al. Field evaluation of anthelmintic drug sensitivity using in vitro egg hatch and larval motility assays with *Necator americanus* recovered from human clinical isolates. *International Journal for Parasitology*, 2005, 35(4):445–453.

257. Kotze AC et al. Dose-response assay templates for in vitro assessment of resistance to benzimidazole and nicotinic acetylcholine receptor agonist drugs in human hookworms. *American Journal of Tropical Medicine and Hygiene*, 2009, 81(1):163–170.

258. Anderson R, May R. *Infectious diseases of humans. Dynamics and control*. Oxford, Oxford University Press, 1992.

259. Chan MS et al. The development and validation of an age-structured model for the evaluation of disease control strategies for intestinal helminths. *Parasitology*, 1994, 109(3):389–396.

260. Anderson RM, May RM. Herd immunity to helminth infection and implications for parasite control. *Nature*, 1985, 315(6019):493–496.

261. Booth M et al. The influence of sampling effort and the performance of the Kato-Katz technique in diagnosing *Schistosoma mansoni* and hookworm co-infections in rural Côte d'Ivoire. *Parasitology*, 2003, 127(6):525–531.

262. Utzinger J et al. Relative contribution of day-to-day and intra-specimen variation in faecal egg counts of *Schistosoma mansoni* before and after treatment with praziquantel. *Parasitology*, 2001, 122(5):537–544.

263. Guyatt H et al. The performance of school-based questionnaires of reported blood in urine in diagnosing *Schistosoma haematobium* infection: patterns by age and sex. *Tropical Medicine & International Health*, 1999, 4(11):751–757.

264. *Report of the WHO Informal Consultation on Schistosomiasis Control, Geneva 2–4 December 1998*. Geneva, World Health Organization, 1999 (http://whqlibdoc.who.int/hq/1999/WHO_CDS_CPC_SIP_99.2.pdf).

265. Doenhoff MJ, Chiodini PL, Hamilton JV. Specific and sensitive diagnosis of schistosome infection: can it be done with antibodies? *Trends in Parasitology*, 2004, 20(1):35–39.

266. McLaren M, Draper CC, Roberts JM. Studies on the enzyme linked immunosorbent assay (ELISA) test for Schistosoma mansoni infections. *Annals of Tropical Medicine and Parasitology*, 1978, 72(3):243–253.

267. Mott KE, Dixon H. Collaborative study on antigens for immunodiagnosis of schistosomiasis. *Bulletin of the World Health Organization*, 1982, 60(5):729–753.

268. Deelder AM et al. *Schistosoma mansoni*: demonstration of two circulating antigens in infected hamsters. *Experimental Parasitology*, 1976, 40(2):189–197.

269. Al-Sherbiny MM et al. Application of immunodiagnostic assays: Detection of antibodies and circulating antigens in human schistosomiasis and correlation with clinical findings. *American Journal of Tropical Medicine and Hygiene*, 1999, 60(6):960–966.

270. Vennervald BJ, Ouma JH, Butterworth AE. Morbidity in schistosomiasis: assessment, mechanisms and control. *Parasitology Today*, 1998, 14(10):385–390.

271. van Dam GJ et al. Diagnosis of schistosomiasis by reagent strip test for detection of circulating cathodic antigen. *Journal of Clinical Microbiology*, 2004, 42(12):5458–5461.

272. Stothard JR et al. Use of circulating cathodic antigen (CCA) dipsticks for detection of intestinal and urinary schistosomiasis. *Acta Tropica*, 2006, 97(2):219–228.

273. ten Hove RJ et al. Multiplex real-time PCR for the detection and quantification of *Schistosoma mansoni* and *S. haematobium* infection in stool samples collected in northern Senegal. *Transactions of the Royal Society of Tropical Medicine and Hygiene*, 2008, 102(2):179–185.

274. Richards CS, Shade PC. The genetic variation of compatibility in *Biomphalaria glabrata* and *Schistosoma mansoni*. *Journal of Parasitology*, 1987, 73(6):1146–1151.

275. Caldeira RL, Jannotti-Passos LK, Carvalho OS. Molecular epidemiology of Brazilian *Biomphalaria*: a review of the identification of species and the detection of infected snails. *Acta Tropica*, 2009, 111(1):1–6.

276. Ismail M et al. Characterization of isolates of *Schistosoma mansoni* from Egyptian villagers that tolerate high doses of praziquantel. *American Journal of Tropical Medicine and Hygiene*, 1996, 55(2):214–218.

277. Gryseels B et al. Epidemiology, immunology and chemotherapy of *Schistosoma mansoni* infections in a recently exposed community in Senegal. *Tropical and Geographical Medicine*, 1994, 46(4):209–219.

278. Stelma FF et al. Morbidity due to heavy *Schistosoma mansoni* infections in a recently established focus in northern Senegal. *American Journal of Tropical Medicine and Hygiene*, 1994, 50(5):575–579.

279. Doenhoff MJ. Is schistosomicidal chemotherapy sub-curative? Implications for drug resistance. *Parasitology Today*, 1998, 14(10):434–435.

280. Steinauer ML et al. Genetic structure of *Schstosoma mansoni* in western Kenya: the effects of geography and host sharing. *International Journal for Parasitology*, 2009, 39(12):1353–1362.

281. Cioli D et al. Determination of ED50 values for praziquantel in praziquantel-resistant and -susceptible *Schistosoma mansoni* isolates. *International Journal for Parasitology*, 2004, 34(8):979–987.

282. Melman SD et al. Reduced susceptibility to praziquantel among naturally occurring Kenyan isolates of *Schistosoma mansoni*. *PLoS Neglected Tropical Diseases*, 2009, 3(8):e504.

283. Liang YS et al. In vitro responses of praziquantel-resistant and -susceptible *Schistosoma mansoni* to praziquantel. *International Journal for Parasitology*, 2001, 31(11):1227–1235.

284. Pica-Mattoccia L, Cioli D. Sex- and stage-related sensitivity of *Schistosoma mansoni* to in vivo and in vitro praziquantel treatment. *International Journal for Parasitology*, 2004, 34(4):527–533.

285. William S, Botros S. Validation of sensitivity to praziquantel using *Schistosoma mansoni* worm muscle tension and Ca2+-uptake as possible in vitro correlates to in vivo ED50 determination. *International Journal for Parasitology*, 2004, 34(8):971–977.

286. Stothard JR et al. The epidemiology and control of urinary schistosomiasis and soil-transmitted helminthiasis in schoolchildren on Unguja Island, Zanzibar. *Transactions of the Royal Society of Tropical Medicine and Hygiene*, 2009, 103(10):1031–1044.

287. Barbour AD. Modeling the transmission of schistosomiasis: an introductory view. *International Journal for Parasitology*, 1996, 55(5 Suppl):135–143.

288. Woolhouse ME. Mathematical models of transmission dynamics and control of schistosomiasis. *American Journal of Tropical Medicine and Hygiene*, 1996, 55(Suppl 5):144–148.

289. Chan MS et al. The development of an age structured model for schistosomiasis transmission dynamics and control and its validation for *Schistosoma mansoni*. *Epidemiology and Infection*, 1995, 115(2):325–344.

290. de Vlas SJ et al. SCHISTOSIM: a microsimulation model for the epidemiology and control of schistosomiasis. *American Journal of Tropical Medicine and Hygiene*, 1996, 55(Suppl 5):170–175.

291. de Vlas SJ et al. A model for variations in single and repeated egg counts in *Schistosoma mansoni* infections. *Parasitology*, 1992, 104(3):451–460.

292. de Vlas SJ et al. Validation of a chart to estimate true *Schistosoma mansoni* prevalences from simple egg counts. *Parasitology*, 1997, 114(2):113–121.

293. Van Lieshout L et al. Analysis of worm burden variation in human *Schistosoma mansoni* infections by determination of serum levels of circulating anodic antigen and circulating cathodic antigen. *Journal of Infectious Diseases*, 1995, 172(5):1336–1342.

294. Polman K et al. Evaluation of density-dependent fecundity in human *Schistosoma mansoni* infections by relating egg counts to circulating antigens through Deming regression. *Parasitology*, 2001, 122(2):161–167.

295. Castillo-Chavez C, Feng Z, Xu D. A schistosomiasis model with mating structure and time delay. *Mathematical Biosciences*, 2008, 211(2):333–341.

296. Feng Z, Curtis J, Minchella DJ. The influence of drug treatment on the maintenance of schistosome genetic diversity. *Journal of Mathematical Biology*, 2001, 43(1):52–68.

297. Xu D et al. On the role of schistosome mating structure in the maintenance of drug resistant strains. *Bulletin of Mathematical Biology*, 2005, 67(6):1207–1226.

298. Wilkins PP et al. Development of a serologic assay to detect *Taenia solium* taeniasis. *American Journal of Tropical Medicine and Hygiene*, 1999, 60(2):199–204.

299. Levine MZ et al. Characterization, cloning, and expression of two diagnostic antigens for *Taenia solium* tapeworm infection. *Journal of Parasitology*, 2004, 90(3):631–638.

300. Allan JC et al. Immunodiagnosis of taeniasis by coproantigen detection. *Parasitology*, 1990, 101(3):473–477.

301. Mayta H et al. Nested PCR for specific diagnosis of *Taenia solium* taeniasis. *Journal of Clinical Microbiology*, 2008, 46(1):286–289.

302. Jeri C et al. Species identification after treatment for human taeniasis. *Lancet*, 2004, 363(9413):949–950.

303. Mahanty S, Garcia HH. Cysticercosis and neurocysticercosis as pathogens affecting the nervous system. *Progress in Neurobiology*, 2010, 91(2):172–184.

304. *Patent royalty rates: a look at recent court decisions*. Adams AF, Calcagno PT, 2008 (http://www.integrityrehab.com/Patent%20Royalty%20Rates%20-%20Recent%20Court%20Decisions%20-%20Adams%204-20-08.pdf, accessed 29 February 2010).

305. Mansfield E, O'Leary TJ, Gutman SI. Food and Drug Administration regulation of in vitro diagnostic devices. *Journal of Molecular Diagnostics*, 2005, 7(1):2–7.

306. MDSS, *In-Vitro Directives Division*, 2011 (http://www.mdss.com/ARServices/IVDD.htm, accessed 29 February 2012).

307. FIND: http://www.finddiagnostics.org/ (accessed 29 February 2012).

308. *A diagnostic path to a better world*. FIND, 2008 (http://www.finddiagnostics.org/export/sites/default/resource-centre/find_documentation/pdfs/diagnostic-path-to-a-better-world.pdf).

309. Habbema JD et al. Epidemiological modelling for onchocerciasis control. *Parasitology Today*, 1992, 8(3):99–103.

310. Koopman J. Modelling infection transmission. *Annual Review of Public Health*, 2004, 25:303–326.

311. Basáñez MG, Ricárdez-Esquinca J. Models for the population biology and control of human onchocerciasis. *Trends in Parasitology*, 2001, 17(9):430–438.

312. Plaisier AP et al. The reproductive lifespan of *Onchocerca volvulus* in West African savanna. *Acta Tropica*, 1991, 48(4):271–284.

313. Fulford AJ et al. A statistical approach to schistosome population dynamics and estimation of the life-span of *Schistosoma mansoni* in man. *Parasitology*, 1995, 110(3):307–316.

314. de Kraker ME et al. Model-based analysis of trial data: microfilaria and worm-productivity loss after diethylcarbamazine-albendazole or ivermectin-albendazole combination therapy against *Wuchereria bancrofti*. *Tropical Medicine & International Health*, 2006, 11(5):718–728.

315. Bottomley C et al. Rates of microfilarial production by *Onchocerca volvulus* are not cumulatively reduced by multiple ivermectin treatments. *Parasitology*, 2008, 135(13):1571–1581.

316. Riley S, Donnelly CA, Ferguson NM. Robust parameter estimation techniques for stochastic within-host macroparasite models. *Journal of Theoretical Biology*, 2003, 225(4):419–430.

317. Brooker S et al. Spatial analysis of the distribution of intestinal nematode infections in Uganda. *Epidemiology and Infection*, 2004, 132(6):1065–1071.

318. Knopp S et al. Spatial distribution of soil-transmitted helminths, including *Strongyloides stercoralis*, among children in Zanzibar. *Geospatial Health*, 2008, 3(1):47–56.

319. Diggle PJ et al. Spatial modelling and the prediction of *Loa loa* risk: decision making under uncertainty. *Annals of Tropical Medicine and Parasitology*, 2007, 101(6):499–509.

320. Clements AC et al. Mapping the probability of schistosomiasis and associated uncertainty, West Africa. *Emerging Infectious Diseases*, 2008, 14(10):1629–1632.

321. Simoonga C et al. Remote sensing, geographical information system and spatial analysis for schistosomiasis epidemiology and ecology in Africa. *Parasitology*, 2009, 136(13):1683–1693.

322. Taylor MJ. *Wolbachia* in the inflammatory pathogenesis of human filariasis. *Annals of the New York Academy of Sciences*, 2003, 990:444–449.

323. Taylor MJ, Bandi C, Hoerauf A. *Wolbachia* bacterial endosymbionts of filarial nematodes. *Advances in Parasitology*, 2005, 60:245–284.

324. Pfarr KM et al. Filariasis and lymphoedema. *Parasite Immunology*, 2009, 31(11):664–672.

325. Murdoch ME et al. A clinical classification and grading system of the cutaneous changes in onchocerciasis. *British Journal of Dermatology*, 1993, 129(3):260–269.

326. Pion SDS et al. Epilepsy in onchocerciasis endemic areas: systematic review and meta-analysis of population-based surveys. *PLoS Neglected Tropical Diseases*, 2009, 3(6):e461.

327. Walker M et al. Density-dependent mortality of the human host in onchocerciasis: Relationships between microfilarial load and excess mortality. *PLoS Neglected Tropical Diseases*, 2012, 6(3):e1578.

328. Savioli L, Albonico M. Soil-transmitted helminthiasis. Nature Reviews *Microbiology*, 2004, 2(8):618–619.

329. Michaud CM, Gordon W, Reich M. *The global burden of disease due to schistosomiasis: Disease Control Priorities Project Working Paper*. Cambridge, Massachusetts, USA, 2003.

330. Vennervald BJ, Polman K. Helminths and malignancy. *Parasite Immunology*, 2009, 31(11):686–696.

331. Sripa B, Pairojkul C. Cholangiocarcinoma: lessons from Thailand. *Current Opinion in Gastroenterology*, 2008, 24(3):349–356.

332. Schistosomes, liver flukes and *Helicobacter pylori*. IARC Working Group on the Evaluation of Carcinogenic Risks to Humans. Lyon, 7–14 June 1994. *IARC Monographs on the Evaluation of Carcinogenic Risks to Humans*, 1994, 61:1–241.

333. Bouvard V et al. A review of human carcinogens – Part B: biological agents. *Lancet Oncology*, 2009, 10(4):321–322.

334. Dietz K. The population dynamics of onchocerciasis. In: Anderson RM ed. *Population dynamics of infectious diseases*. London: Chapman and Hall, 1982:209–241.

335. Basáñez MG, Boussinesq M. Population biology of human onchocerciasis. *Philosophical Transactions of the Royal Society of London. Series B, Biological Sciences*, 1999, 354:809–826.

336. Basáñez MG et al. Transmission intensity and the patterns of *Onchocerca volvulus* infection in human communities. *American Journal of Tropical Medicine and Hygiene*, 2002, 67(6):669–679.

337. Duerr HP, Eichner M. Epidemiology and control of onchocerciasis: the threshold biting rate of savannah onchocerciasis in Africa. *International Journal for Parasitology*, 2009, 40(6):641–650.

338. Churcher TS, Filipe JA, Basáñez MG. Density dependence and the control of helminth parasites. *Journal of Animal Ecology*, 2006, 75(6):1313–1320.

339. Duerr HP, Dietz K, Eichner M. Determinants of the eradicability of filarial infections: a conceptual approach. *Trends in Parasitology*, 2005, 21(2):88–96.

340. Saathoff E et al. Patterns of geohelminth infection, impact of albendazole treatment and re-infection after treatment in schoolchildren from rural KwaZulu-Natal/South-Africa. *BMC Infectious Diseases*, 2004, 4:27.

341. Raso G et al. Multiple parasite infections and their relationship to self-reported morbidity in a community of rural Côte d'Ivoire. *International Journal of Epidemiology*, 2004, 33(5):1092–1102.

342. Brooker S et al. Epidemiology of *Plasmodium*-helminth co-infection in Africa: populations at risk, potential impact on anemia, and prospects for combining control. *American Journal of Tropical Medicine and Hygiene*, 2007, 77(Suppl 6):88–98.

343. Pion SD et al. Co-infection with *Onchocerca volvulus* and *Loa loa* microfilariae in central Cameroon: are these two species interacting? *Parasitology*, 2006, 132(6):843–854.

344. Pullan R, Brooker S. The health impact of polyparasitism in humans: are we under-estimating the burden of parasitic diseases? *Parasitology*, 2008, 135(7):783–794.

345. Pullan RL et al. Human helminth co-infection: analysis of spatial patterns and risk factors in a Brazilian community. *PLoS Neglected Tropical Diseases*, 2008, 2(12):e352.

346. Liang S et al. Re-emerging schistosomiasis in hilly and mountainous areas of Sichuan, China. *Bulletin of the World Health Organization*, 2006, 84(2):139–144.

347. Sousa-Figueiredo JC et al. A parasitological survey, in rural Zanzibar, of pre-school children and their mothers for urinary schistosomiasis, soil-transmitted helminthiases and malaria, with observations on the prevalence of anaemia. *Annals of Tropical Medicine and Parasitology*, 2008, 102(8):679–692.

348. Brooker S et al. Evaluating the epidemiological impact of national control programmes for helminths. *Trends in Parasitology*, 2004, 20(11):537–545.

349. Guyatt HL et al. The relationship between the frequency distribution of *Ascaris lumbricoides* and the prevalence and intensity of infection in human communities. *Parasitology*, 1990, 101(1):139–143.

350. Mukoko DA et al. Bancroftian filariasis in 12 villages in Kwale district, Coast province, Kenya - variation in clinical and parasitological patterns. *Annals of Tropical Medicine and Parasitology*, 2004, 98(8):801–815.

351. Rudge JW et al. Micro-epidemiology of urinary schistosomiasis in Zanzibar: Local risk factors associated with distribution of infections among schoolchildren and relevance for control. *Acta Tropica*, 2008, 105(1):45–54.

352. Tarafder MR et al. A cross-sectional study of the prevalence of intensity of infection with *Schistosoma japonicum* in 50 irrigated and rain-fed villages in Samar Province, the Philippines. *BMC Public Health*, 2006, 6:61.

353. Churcher TS, Ferguson NM, Basáñez MG. Density dependence and overdispersion in the transmission of helminth parasites. *Parasitology*, 2005, 131(1):121–132.

354. Huppatz C et al. Lessons from the Pacific programme to eliminate lymphatic filariasis: a case study of 5 countries. *BMC Infectious Diseases*, 2009, 9:92.

355. Knopp S et al. Changing patterns of soil-transmitted helminthiases in Zanzibar in the context of national helminth control programs. *American Journal of Tropical Medicine and Hygiene*, 2009, 81(6):1071–1078.

356. Bottomley C, Isham V, Basáñez MG. Population biology of multispecies helminth infection: interspecific interactions and parasite distribution. *Parasitology*, 2005, 131(3):417–433.

357. Fenton A. Worms and germs: the population dynamic consequences of microparasite-macroparasite co-infection. *Parasitology*, 2008, 135(13):1545–1560.

358. Fenton A, Lamb T, Graham AL. Optimality analysis of Th1/Th2 immune responses during microparasite-macroparasite co-infection, with epidemiological feedbacks. *Parasitology*, 2008, 135(7):841–853.

359. Lello J et al. Pathogen interactions, population cycles, and phase shifts. *American Naturalist*, 2008, 171(2):176–182.

360. Gurarie D, King CH. Heterogeneous model of schistosomiasis transmission and long-term control: the combined influence of spatial variation and age-dependent factors on optimal allocation of drug therapy. *Parasitology*, 2005, 130(1):49–65.

361. Gurarie D, Seto EY. Connectivity sustains disease transmission in environments with low potential for endemicity: modelling schistosomiasis with hydrologic and social connectivities. *Journal of the Royal Society Interface*, 2009, 6(35):495–508.

362. Waghorn TS et al. Brave or gullible: testing the concept that leaving susceptible parasites in refugia will slow the development of anthelmintic resistance. *New Zealand Veterinary Journal*, 2008, 56(4):158–163.

363. Anderson RM, May RM. Helminth infections of humans: mathematical models, population dynamics, and control. *Advances in Parasitology*, 1985, 24:1–101.

364. Woolhouse ME. On the application of mathematical models of schistosome transmission dynamics. I. Natural transmission. *Acta Tropica*, 1991, 49(4):241–270.

365. Duerr HP et al. The relationships between the burden of adult parasites, host age and the microfilarial density in human onchocerciasis. *International Journal for Parasitology*, 2004, 34(4):463–473.

366. Duerr HP et al. Density-dependent parasite establishment suggests infection-associated immunosuppression as an important mechanism for parasite density regulation in onchocerciasis. *Transactions of the Royal Society of Tropical Medicine and Hygiene*, 2003, 97(2):242–250.

367. Filipe JA et al. Human infection patterns and heterogeneous exposure in river blindness. *Proceedings of the National Academy of Sciences of the United States of America*, 2005, 102(42):15265–15270.

368. Plaisier AP et al. ONCHOSIM: a model and computer simulation program for the transmission and control of onchocerciasis. *Computer Methods and Programs in Biomedicine*, 1990, 31(1):43–56.

369. Plaisier AP et al. Required duration of combined annual ivermectin treatment and vector control in the Onchocerciasis Control Programme in West Africa. *Bulletin of the World Health Organization*, 1997, 75(3):237–245.

370. Winnen M et al. Can ivermectin mass treatments eliminate onchocerciasis in Africa? *Bulletin of the World Health Organization*, 2002, 80(5):384–391.

371. Woolhouse ME. On the application of mathematical models of schistosome transmission dynamics. II. Control. *Acta Tropica*, 1992, 50(3):189–204.

372. Woolhouse ME. Human schistosomiasis: potential consequences of vaccination. *Vaccine*, 1995, 13(12):1045–1050.

373. Chan MS, Woolhouse ME, Bundy DAP. Human schistosomiasis: potential long-term consequences of vaccination programmes. *Vaccine*, 1997, 15(14):1545–1550.

374. Chan MS et al. Epifil: a dynamic model of infection and disease in lymphatic filariasis. *American Journal of Tropical Medicine and Hygiene*, 1998, 59(4):606–614.

375. Norman RA et al. EPIFIL: the development of an age-structured model for describing the transmission dynamics and control of lymphatic filariasis. *Epidemiology and Infection*, 2000, 124(3):529–541.

376. Michael E et al. Mathematical models and lymphatic filariasis control: endpoints and optimal interventions. *Trends in Parasitology*, 2006, 22(5):226–233.

377. Kyvsgaard NC, Johansen MV, Carabin H. Simulating transmission and control of *Taenia solium* infections using a Reed-Frost stochastic model. *International Journal for Parasitology*, 2007, 37(5):547–558.

378. Torgerson PR. Mathematical models for the control of cystic echinococcosis. *Parasitology International*, 2006, 55(Suppl):S253–258.

379. Roberts MG, Lawson JR, Gemmell MA. Population dynamics in echinococcosis and cysticercosis: mathematical model of the life-cycles of *Taenia hydatigena* and *T. ovis*. *Parasitology*, 1987, 94(1):181–197.

380. Roberts MG. Modelling of parasitic populations: cestodes. *Veterinary Parasitology*, 1994, 54(1-3):145–160.

381. Brindley PJ et al. Helminth genomics: The implications for human health. *PLoS Neglected Tropical Diseases*, 2009, 3(10):e538.

382. Abubucker S et al. The canine hookworm genome: analysis and classification of *Ancylostoma caninum* survey sequences. *Molecular and Biochemical Parasitology*, 2008, 157(2):187–192.

383. Zhou Y et al. The *Schistosoma japonicum* genome reveals features of host-parasite interplay. *Nature*, 2009, 460(7253):345–351.

384. Brindley PJ. The molecular biology of schistosomes. *Trends in Parasitology*, 2005, 21(11):533–536.

385. Malaria Drug Targets (MDT). *A malarial target and inhibitor database*, 2011 (http://www.bioinformatics.org/mdt, accessed 2 March 2012).

386. WHO Special Programme for Research and Training in Tropical Diseases (TDR). *The TDR Targets Database v4: A chemogenomics resource for neglected tropical diseases*. TDR, 2011 (http://www.tdrtargets.org/, accessed 2 March 2012).

387. Aguero F et al. Genomic-scale prioritization of drug targets: the TDR Targets database. *Nature Reviews Drug Discovery*, 2008, 7(11):900–907.

388. Spiliotis M et al. Transient transfection of *Echinococcus multilocularis* primary cells and complete in vitro regeneration of metacestode vesicles. *International Journal for Parasitology*, 2008, 38(8-9):1025–1039.

389. Gobert GN et al. Transcriptomics tool for the human *Schistosoma* blood flukes using microarray gene expression profiling. *Experimental Parasitology*, 2006, 114(3):160–172.

390. Dillon GP et al. Patterns of gene expression in schistosomes: localization by whole mount in situ hybridization. *Parasitology*, 2007, 134(11):1589–1597.

391. Hewitson JP, Grainger JR, Maizels RM. Helminth immunoregulation: the role of parasite secreted proteins in modulating host immunity. *Molecular and Biochemical Parasitology*, 2009, 167(1):1–11.

392. Nacher M et al. Intestinal helminth infections are associated with increased incidence of *Plasmodium falciparum* malaria in Thailand. *Journal of Parasitology*, 2002, 88(1):55–58.

393. Nacher M. Malaria vaccine trials in a wormy world. *Trends in Parasitology*, 2001, 17(12):563–565.

394. Druilhe P, Tall A, Sokhna C. Worms can worsen malaria: towards a new means to roll back malaria? *Trends in Parasitology*, 2005, 21(8):359–362.

395. Murray MJ et al. Parotid enlargement, forehead edema, and suppression of malaria as nutritional consequences of ascariasis. *American Journal of Clinical Nutrition*, 1977, 30(12):2117–2121.

396. Murray J et al. The biological suppression of malaria: an ecological and nutritional interrelationship of a host and two parasites. *American Journal of Clinical Nutrition*, 1978, 31(8):1363–1366.

397. Schijns VE. Immunological concepts of vaccine adjuvant activity. *Current Opinion in Immunology*, 2000, 12(4):456–463.

398. Cooper PJ et al. Impaired tetanus-specific cellular and humoral responses following tetanus vaccination in human onchocerciasis: a possible role for interleukin-10. *Journal of Infectious Diseases*, 1998, 178(4):1133–1138.

399. Cooper PJ et al. Human infection with *Ascaris lumbricoides* is associated with a polarized cytokine response. *Journal of Infectious Diseases*, 2000, 182(4):1207–1213.

400. Sabin EA et al. Impairment of tetanus toxoid-specific Th1-like immune responses in humans infected with *Schistosoma mansoni*. *Journal of Infectious Diseases*, 1996, 173(1):269–272.

401. Cooper PJ et al. Human infection with *Ascaris lumbricoides* is associated with suppression of the interleukin-2 response to recombinant cholera toxin B subunit following vaccination with the live oral cholera vaccine CVD 103-HgR. *Infection and Immunity*, 2001, 69(3):1574–1580.

402. Hatherill M et al. The potential impact of helminth infection on trials of novel tuberculosis vaccines. *Vaccine*, 2009, 27(35):4743–4744.

403. Cruz-Chan JV, Rosado-Vallado M, Dumonteil E. Malaria vaccine efficacy: overcoming the helminth hurdle. *Expert Review of Vaccines*, 2010, 9(7):707–711.

404. Duke BOL, Moore PJ. The contributions of different age groups to the transmission of onchocerciasis in a Cameroon forest village. *Transactions of the Royal Society of Tropical Medicine and Hygiene*, 1968, 62(1):22–28.

405. Abraham D, Lucius R, Trees AJ. Immunity to *Onchocerca* spp. in animal hosts. *Trends in Parasitology*, 2002, 18(4):164–171.

406. Njongmeta LM et al. Cattle protected from onchocerciasis by ivermectin are highly susceptible to infection after drug withdrawal. *International Journal for Parasitology*, 2004, 34(9):1069–1074.

407. Maizels RM et al. Regulation of pathogenesis and immunity in helminth infections. *Journal of Experimental Medicine*, 2009, 206(10):2059–2066.

408. Shaw MA, Quinnell RJ. Human genetics and resistance to parasitic infection. *Parasite Immunology*, 2009, 31(5):221–224.

409. Mas-Coma S, Valero MA, Bargues MD. Fasciola, lymnaeids and human fascioliasis, with a global overview on disease transmission, epidemiology, evolutionary genetics, molecular epidemiology and control. *Advances in Parasitology*, 2009, 69:41–146.

410. Rim HJ. Clonorchiasis: an update. *Journal of Helminthology*, 2005, 79(3):269–281.

411. Sripa B. Pathobiology of opisthorchiasis: an update. *Acta Tropica*, 2003, 88(3):209–220.

412. Robinson MW et al. An integrated transcriptomics and proteomics analysis of the secretome of the helminth pathogen *Fasciola hepatica*: proteins associated with invasion and infection of the mammalian host. *Molecular & Cellular Proteomics*, 2009, 8(8):1891–1907.

413. Kim YJ et al. Proliferative effects of excretory/secretory products from Clonorchis sinensis on the human epithelial cell line HEK293 via regulation of the transcription factor E2F1. *Parasitology Research*, 2008, 102(3):411–417.

414. Thuwajit C et al. Increased cell proliferation of mouse fibroblast NIH-3T3 in vitro induced by excretory/secretory product(s) from *Opisthorchis viverrini*. *Parasitology*, 2004, 129(4):455–464.

415. Bennuru S, Nutman TB. Lymphangiogenesis and lymphatic remodeling induced by filarial parasites: implications for pathogenesis. *PLoS Pathogens*, 2009, 5(12):e1000688.

416. Freedman DO, Ottesen EA. Eggs of *Schistosoma mansoni* stimulate endothelial cell proliferation in vitro. *Journal of Infectious Diseases*, 1988, 158(3):556–562.

417. Bennuru S et al. *Brugia malayi* excreted/secreted proteins at the host/parasite interface: stage- and gender-specific proteomic profiling. *PLoS Neglected Tropical Diseases*, 2009, 3(4):e410.

418. Higazi TB et al. *Wolbachia* endosymbiont levels in severe and mild strains of *Onchocerca volvulus*. *Molecular and Biochemical Parasitology*, 2005, 141(1):109–112.

419. Griffin JT et al. Reducing *Plasmodium falciparum* malaria transmission in Africa: a model-based evaluation of intervention strategies. *PLoS Medicine*, 2010, 7(8):e1000324.

420. Shriram AN et al. Diurnal pattern of human-biting activity and transmission of subperiodic *Wuchereria bancrofti* (Filarioidea: Dipetalonematidae) by *Ochlerotatus niveus* (Diptera: Culicidae) on the Andaman and Nicobar islands of India. *American Journal of Tropical Medicine and Hygiene*, 2005, 72(3):273–277.

421. Bockarie MJ et al. Role of vector control in the global program to eliminate lymphatic filariasis. *Annual Review of Entomology*, 2009, 54:469–487.

422. Haas W et al. Finding and recognition of the snail intermediate hosts by 3 species of echinostome cercariae. *Parasitology*, 1995, 110(2):133–142.

423. Kalbe M et al. Heredity of specific host-finding behaviour in *Schistosoma mansoni* miracidia. *Parasitology*, 2004, 128(6):635–643.

424. Sukhdeo MVK, Sukhdeo SC. Trematode behaviours and the perceptual worlds of parasites. *Canadian Journal of Zoology*, 2004, 82:292–315.

425. Gower CM, Webster JP. Fitness of indirectly transmitted pathogens: restraint and constraint. *Evolution*, 2004, 58(6):1178–1184.

426. Hassan AH et al. Miracidia of an Egyptian strain of *Schistosoma mansoni* differentiate between sympatric snail species. *Journal of Parasitology*, 2003, 89(6):1248–1250.

427. Kalbe M, Haberl B, Haas W. *Schistosoma mansoni* miracidial host-finding: species specificity of an Egyptian strain. *Parasitology Research*, 1996, 82(1):8–13.

428. Davies CM, Fairbrother E, Webster JP. Mixed strain schistosome infections of snails and the evolution of parasite virulence. *Parasitology*, 2002, 124(1):31–38.

429. Norton A et al. Simultaneous infection of *Schistosoma mansoni* and *S. rodhaini* in *Biomphalaria glabrata*: impact on chronobiology and cercarial behaviour. *Parasites & Vectors*, 2008, 1(1):43.

430. Lu DB et al. Evolution in a multi-host parasite: chronobiological circadian rhythm and population genetics of *Schistosoma japonicum* cercariae indicates contrasting definitive host reservoirs by habitat. *International Journal for Parasitology*, 2009, 39(14):1581–1588.

431. Botros S et al. Current status of sensitivity to praziquantel in a focus of potential drug resistance in Egypt. *International Journal for Parasitology*, 2005, 35(7):787–791.

432. Pinlaor S et al. Oxidative and nitrative stress in *Opisthorchis viverrini*-infected hamsters: an indirect effect after praziquantel treatment. *American Journal of Tropical Medicine and Hygiene*, 2008, 78(4):564–573.

433. Pinlaor S et al. Repeated infection with *Opisthorchis viverrini* induces accumulation of 8-nitroguanine and 8-oxo-7,8-dihydro-2'-deoxyguanine in the bile duct of hamsters via inducible nitric oxide synthase. *Carcinogenesis*, 2004, 25(8):1535–1542.

434. Taylor MJ, Hoerauf A. *Wolbachia* bacteria of filarial nematodes. *Parasitology Today*, 1999, 15(11):437–442.

435. Bandi C, Trees AJ, Brattig NW. *Wolbachia* in filarial nematodes: evolutionary aspects and implications for the pathogenesis and treatment of filarial diseases. *Veterinary Parasitology*, 2001, 98(1-3):215–238.

436. Selkirk ME, Maizels RM, Yazdanbakhsh M. Immunity and the prospects for vaccination against filariasis. *Immunobiology*, 1992, 184(2-3):263–281.

437. Brattig NW et al. Lipopolysaccharide-like molecules derived from *Wolbachia* endobacteria of the filaria *Onchocerca volvulus* are candidate mediators in the sequence of inflammatory and antiinflammatory responses of human monocytes. *Microbes and Infection*, 2000, 2(10):1147–1157.

438. Taylor MJ, Cross HF, Bilo K. Inflammatory responses induced by the filarial nematode *Brugia malayi* are mediated by lipopolysaccharide-like activity from endosymbiotic *Wolbachia* bacteria. *Journal of Experimental Medicine*, 2000, 191(8):1429–1436.

439. Brattig NW, Buttner DW, Hoerauf A. Neutrophil accumulation around *Onchocerca* worms and chemotaxis of neutrophils are dependent on *Wolbachia* endobacteria. *Microbes and Infection*, 2001, 3(6):439–446.

440. Brattig NW et al. The major surface protein of *Wolbachia* endosymbionts in filarial nematodes elicits immune responses through TLR2 and TLR4. *Journal of Immunology*, 2004, 173(1):437–445.

441. Cross HF et al. Severe reactions to filarial chemotherapy and release of *Wolbachia* endosymbionts into blood. *Lancet*, 2001, 358(9296):1873–1875.

442. Keiser PB et al. Bacterial endosymbionts of *Onchocerca volvulus* in the pathogenesis of posttreatment reactions. *Journal of Infectious Diseases*, 2002, 185(6):805–811.

443. Saint André A et al. The role of endosymbiotic *Wolbachia* bacteria in the pathogenesis of river blindness. *Science*, 2002, 295(5561):1892–1895.

444. Semnani RT, Nutman TB. Toward an understanding of the interaction between filarial parasites and host antigen-presenting cells. *Immunological Reviews*, 2004, 201:127–138.

445. Nutman TB et al. Immunity to onchocerciasis: recognition of larval antigens by humans putatively immune to *Onchocerca volvulus* infection. *Journal of Infectious Diseases*, 1991, 163(5):1128–1133.

446. Lustigman S, MacDonald AJ, Abraham D. CD4+ dependent immunity to *Onchocerca volvulus* third-stage larvae in humans and the mouse vaccination model: common ground and distinctions. *International Journal for Parasitology*, 2003, 33(11):1161–1171.

447. MacDonald AJ et al. Differential cytokine and antibody responses to adult and larval stages of *Onchocerca volvulus* consistent with the development of concomitant immunity. *Infection and Immunity*, 2002, 70(6):2796–2804.
448. Andrade ZA. Schistosomiasis and liver fibrosis. *Parasite Immunology*, 2009, 31(11):656–663.
449. Burke ML et al. Immunopathogenesis of human schistosomiasis. *Parasite Immunology*, 2009, 31(4):163–176.
450. Blanton RE et al. Schistosomal hepatic fibrosis and the interferon gamma receptor: a linkage analysis using single-nucleotide polymorphic markers. *European Journal of Human Genetics*, 2005, 13(5):660–668.
451. Campino S, Kwiatkowski D, Dessein A. Mendelian and complex genetics of susceptibility and resistance to parasitic infections. *Semininars in Immunology*, 2006, 18(6):411–422.
452. Dessein AJ et al. Severe hepatic fibrosis in *Schistosoma mansoni* infection is controlled by a major locus that is closely linked to the interferon-gamma receptor gene. *American Journal of Human Genetics*, 1999, 65(3):709–721.
453. Marquet S et al. Full results of the genome-wide scan which localises a locus controlling the intensity of infection by *Schistosoma mansoni* on chromosome 5q31-q33. *European Journal of Human Genetics*, 1999, 7(1):88–97.
454. Marquet S et al. Genetic localization of a locus controlling the intensity of infection by *Schistosoma mansoni* on chromosome 5q31-q33. *Nature Genetics*, 1996, 14(2):181–184.
455. Sripa B et al. Advanced periductal fibrosis from infection with the carcinogenic human liver fluke *Opisthorchis viverrini* correlates with elevated levels of interleukin-6. *Hepatology*, 2009, 50(4):1273–1281.
456. Garcia HH, Del Brutto OH. Neurocysticercosis: updated concepts about an old disease. *Lancet Neurology*, 2005, 4(10):653–661.
457. Sinha S, Sharma BS. Neurocysticercosis: a review of current status and management. *Journal of Clinical Neuroscience*, 2009, 16(7):867–876.
458. Prasad KN et al. Human cysticercosis and Indian scenario: a review. *Journal of Biosciences*, 2008, 33(4):571–582.
459. Aguilar-Diaz H et al. The genome project of *Taenia solium*. *Parasitology International*, 2006, 55 Suppl:S127–130.
460. Campbell G et al. Genetic variation in *Taenia solium*. *Parasitology International*, 2006, 55(Suppl):S121–S126.
461. Sciutto E et al. The immune response in *Taenia solium* cysticercosis: protection and injury. *Parasite Immunology*, 2007, 29(12):621–636.
462. Terrazas LI. The complex role of pro- and anti-inflammatory cytokines in cysticercosis: immunological lessons from experimental and natural hosts. *Current Topics in Medical Chemistry*, 2008, 8(5):383–392.
463. *Community-directed interventions for major health problems in Africa. A multi-country study*. Geneva, World Health Organization, 2008.
464. *Community participation and tropical disease control in resource-poor settings*. Geneva, World Health Organization, 2004.
465. Theobald S, Tolhurst R, Squire SB. Gender, equity: new approaches for effective management of communicable diseases. *Transactions of the Royal Society of Tropical Medicine and Hygiene*, 2006, 100(4):299–304.

466. Renz A, Fuglsang H, Anderson J. Studies on the dynamics of transmission of onchocerciasis in a Sudan-savanna area of North Cameroon IV. The different exposure to *Simulium* bites and transmission of boys and girls and men and women, and the resulting manifestations of onchocerciasis. *Annals of Tropical Medicine and Parasitology*, 1987, 81(3):253–262.

467. Braga C et al. Bancroftian filariasis in an endemic area of Brazil: differences between genders during puberty. *Revista da Sociedade Brasileira de Medicina Tropical*, 2005, 38(3):224–228.

468. Vlassoff C et al. Gender and the stigma of onchocercal skin disease in Africa. *Social Science & Medicine*, 2000, 50(10):1353–1368.

469. Babu BV et al. Knowledge and beliefs about elephantiasis and hydrocele of lymphatic filariasis and some socio-demographic determinants in an endemic community of Eastern India. *Public Health*, 2004, 118(2):121–127.

470. Clemmons L et al. Gender issues in the community-directed treatment with ivermectin (CDTI) of the African Programme for Onchocerciasis Control (APOC). *Annals of Tropical Medicine and Parasitology*, 2002, 96(Suppl 1):S59–S74.

471. Wani SA, Ahmad F. Intestinal helminths and associated risk factors in children of district Pulwama, Kashmir, India. *Indian Journal of Medical Microbiology*, 2009, 27(1):81–82.

472. Heijnders ML. The dynamics of stigma in leprosy. *International Journal of Leprosy and Other Mycobacterial Diseases*, 2004, 72(4):437–447.

473. McMichael AJ et al., eds. *Climate change and human health: risk and responses*. Geneva, World Health Organization, 2003.

474. Patz JA et al. Impact of regional climate change on human health. *Nature*, 2005, 438(7066):310–317.

475. Ezzati M et al. Environmental risks in the developing world: exposure indicators for evaluating interventions, programmes, and policies. *Journal of Epidemiology and Community Health*, 2005, 59(1):15–22.

476. Reiter P. Climate change and mosquito-borne disease. *Environmental Health Perspectives*, 2001, 109(Suppl 1):141–161.

477. Hunter PR. Climate change and waterborne and vector-borne disease. *Journal of Applied Microbiology*, 2003, 94(Suppl):S37–S46.

478. Sutherst RW. Global change and human vulnerability to vector-borne diseases. *Clinical Microbiology Reviews*, 2004, 17(1):136–173.

479. Patz JA et al. Effects of environmental change on emerging parasitic diseases. *International Journal for Parasitology*, 2000, 30(12-3):1395–1405.

480. Morgan ER, Wall R. Climate change and parasitic disease: farmer mitigation? *Trends in Parasitology*, 2009, 25(7):308–313.

481. Yang GJ et al. A potential impact of climate change and water resource development on the transmission of *Schistosoma japonicum* in China. *Parassitologia*, 2005, 47(1):127–134.

482. Yang GJ et al. Remote sensing for predicting potential habitats of *Oncomelania hupensis* in Hongze, Baima and Gaoyou lakes in Jiangsu province, China. *Geospatial Health*, 2006, 1(1):85–92.

483. Zhou XN et al. Potential impact of climate change on schistosomiasis transmission in China. *American Journal of Tropical Medicine and Hygiene*, 2008, 78(2):188–194.

484. Mangal TD, Paterson S, Fenton A. Predicting the impact of long-term temperature changes on the epidemiology and control of schistosomiasis: a mechanistic model. *PLoS ONE*, 2008, 3(1):e1438.

485. Xu XJ et al. Impact of environmental change and schistosomiasis transmission in the middle reaches of the Yangtze River following the Three Gorges construction project. *Southeast Asian Journal of Tropical Medicine and Public Health*, 1999, 30(3):549–555.

486. Xu XJ et al. Possible effects of the Three Gorges dam on the transmission of *Schistosoma japonicum* on the Jiang Han plain, China. *Annals of Tropical Medicine and Parasitology*, 2000, 94(4):333–341.

487. Spiegel A et al. Increased frequency of malaria attacks in subjects co-infected by intestinal worms and *Plasmodium falciparum* malaria. *Transactions of the Royal Society of Tropical Medicine and Hygiene*, 2003, 97(2):198–199.

488. Le Hesran JY et al. Severe malaria attack is associated with high prevalence of *Ascaris lumbricoides* infection among children in rural Senegal. *Transactions of the Royal Society of Tropical Medicine and Hygiene*, 2004, 98(7):397–399.

489. Mwatha JK et al. Associations between anti-*Schistosoma mansoni* and anti-*Plasmodium falciparum* antibody responses and hepatosplenomegaly, in Kenyan schoolchildren. *Journal of Infectious Diseases*, 2003, 187(8):1337–1341.

490. Bockarie MJ, Taylor MJ, Gyapong JO. Current practices in the management of lymphatic filariasis. *Expert Review of Anti-Infective Therapy*, 2009, 7(5):595–605.

491. Ramaiah KD et al. Effectiveness of community and health services-organized drug delivery strategies for elimination of lymphatic filariasis in rural areas of Tamil Nadu, India. *Tropical Medicine & International Health*, 2001, 6(12):1062–1069.

492. WHO. Global programme to eliminate lymphatic filariasis. *Weekly Epidemiological Record*, 2010, 85(38):365–372.

493. Volmink J, Dare L. Addressing inequalities in research capacity in Africa. *British Medical Journal*, 2005, 331(7519):705–706.

494. Wagner CS et al. *Science and technology collaboration: building capacity in developing countries?* USA, RAND Science and Technology, 2001 (http://www.rand.org/pubs/monograph_reports/2005/MR1357.0.pdf).

495. Chauhan R. Lack of research impetus in Africa: a way forward. Rapid responses to addressing inequalities in research capacity in Africa. *British Medical Journal*, 2005, 331:705–706.

496. Lustigman S et al. A research agenda for helminth diseases of humans: The problem of helminthiases. *PLoS Neglected Tropical Diseases*, 2012, 6(4):e1582.

497. Prichard RK et al. A research agenda for helminth diseases of humans: Intervention for control and elimination. *PLoS Neglected Tropical Diseases*, 2012, 6(4):e1549.

498. Gazzinelli A et al. A research agenda for helminth diseases of humans: Social ecology, environmental determinants and health systems. *PLoS Neglected Tropical Diseases*, 2012, 6(4):e1603.

499. Colley DG, LoVerde PT, Savioli L. Infectious disease. Medical helminthology in the 21st century. *Science*, 2001, 293(5534):1437–1438.

500. Boatin BA et al. A research agenda for helminth diseases of humans: Towards control and elimination. *PLoS Neglected Tropical Diseases*, 2012, 6(4):e1547.

501. Conteh L, Engels T, Molyneux DH. Socioeconomic aspects of neglected tropical diseases. *Lancet*, 2010, 375(9710):239–247.

502. Savino W et al. Local generation of high-quality human resources for health research. *Bulletin of the World Health Organization*, 2008, 86(12):910.

503. Almeida C et al. Brazil's conception of South-South "structural cooperation" in health. *Revista Eletrônica de Comunicação Informação & Inovação em Saúde*, Rio de Janeiro, 2010, 4:23–32.

504. Moran M et al. Neglected disease research and development: how much are we really spending? *PLoS Medicine*, 2009, 6(2):e30.

505. *Capacity building in Africa. An OED evaluation of World Bank support*. Washington, The World Bank, Operations Evaluation Department, 2005 (http://www.worldbank.org/oed/africa_capacity_building, accessed 2 March 2012).

506. Healthlink. Communicating health research: how should evidence affect policy and practice? Stronger links between researchers, policy makers and practitioners and increased southern research capacity are the keys to relevant evidence being taken up. *Findings*, 2006, 5 (http://www.healthlink.org.uk/PDFs/findings_research.pdf).

507. Basáñez MG et al. A research agenda for helminth diseases of humans: modelling for control and elimination. *PLoS Neglected Tropical Diseases*, 2012, 6(4)e1548.

508. Kariuki T et al. Research and capacity building for control of neglected tropical diseases: the need for a different approach. *PLoS Neglected Tropical Diseases*, 2011, 5(5):e1020.

509. Overview and report from the Algiers preparatory meeting, and report from other preparatory meetings related to the Bamako Call for Action. In: *Global Ministerial Forum on Research for Health*, 2008 (http://www.tropika.net/svc/specials/bamako2008/session-reports/ministerial-discussions-day-1, accessed 2 March 2012).

510. Wilder R, Solovy EM. *The development of medicines for developing country diseases: the role of intellectual property*. World Intellectual Property Organization, 2005 (http://www.wipo.int/edocs/mdocs/mdocs/en/isipd_05/isipd_05_www_103972.pdf, accessed 2 March 2012).

511. *Civil society report on intellectual property, innovation and health*. IPN, 2006 (http://www.policynetwork.net/es/health/publication/civil-society-report-intellectual-property-innovation-health, accessed 2 March 2012).

512. Degrave W et al. *Bioinformatics for disease endemic countries: opportunities and challenges in science and technology development for health*. Special Programme for Research and Training in Tropical Diseases (TDR), 2002 (http://www.ibioseminars.org/roos/TDRbioinformatics.pdf, accessed 2 March 2012).

513. Nashiru O et al. Building bioinformatics capacity in West Africa. *African Journal of Medicine and Medical Sciences*, 2007, 36 Suppl:15–18.

514. *Global plan to combat neglected tropical diseases 2008–2015*. World Health Organization, 2007 (http://whqlibdoc.who.int/hq/2007/who_cds_ntd_2007.3_eng.pdf, accessed 2 March 2012).

515. Morel CM et al. Health innovation networks to help developing countries address neglected diseases. *Science*, 2005, 309(5733):401–404.

516. Hotez PJ et al. Hookworm: "the great infection of mankind". *PLoS Medicine*, 2005, 2(3):e67.

517. Xiao S et al. Recent investigations of artemether, a novel agent for the prevention of schistosomiasis japonica, mansoni and haematobia. *Acta Tropica*, 2002, 82(2):175–181.

518. Grace C. *The effect of changing intellectual property on pharmaceutical industry prospects in India and China: Considerations for access to medicine*. Issues Paper, Health Systems Resource Centre, United Kingdom Department for International Development (DfID), 2004 (http://www.who.int/hiv/amds/Grace2China.pdf, accessed 2 March 2012).

519. Tanner M, Kitua A, Degremont AA. Developing health research capability in Tanzania: from a Swiss Tropical Institute Field Laboratory to the Ifakara Centre of the Tanzanian National Institute of Medical Research. *Acta Tropica*, 1994, 57(2-3):153–173.

520. Ofori-Adjei D. Investing in health research for endemic diseases. *Ghana Medical Journal*, 2008, 42(3):95.

521. Bonfoh B et al. Research in a war zone. *Nature*, 2011, 474(7353):569–571.

522. *Guidelines for research in partnership with developing countries. 11 Principles*. Swiss Commission for Research Partnerships with Developing Countries, KFPE, Swiss Academy of Sciences, 1998 (http://www.kfpe.ch/download/Guidelines_e.pdf, accessed 2 March 2012).

523. *Guidelines for research in partnership with developing countries: 12 principles*. Swiss Commission for Research Partnerships with Developing Countries, KFPE Swiss Academy of Sciences, 2000.

524. Ofori-Adjei D, Gyapong J. *A developing country perspective on international research partnerships on health*. Netherlands Organisation for International Cooperation in Higher Education, 2008 (http://www.nuffic.nl/home/news-events/docs/events/kotm/abstracts-and-papers/International%20Research%20Partnerships%20on%20Health%20Final.pdf, accessed 2 March 2012).

525. Bethony JM, Loukas A. The schistosomiasis research agenda – what now? *PLoS Neglected Tropical Diseases*, 2008, 2(2):e207.

526. Young J, Kannemeyer N. *Building capacity in Southern research: A study to map existing initiatives. Main Report*. London, Overseas Development Institute (DfID), 2001 (http://www.odi.org.uk/resources/download/2845.pdf:).

527. Binka F. Editorial. North-south research collaborations: a move towards a true partnership? *Tropical Medicine & International Health*, 2005, 10(3):207–209.

528. *Abuja Declaration on HIV/AIDS. Tuberculosis and other related infectious diseases*. Abuja, Nigeria, 2001 (http://www.un.org/ga/aids/pdf/abuja_declaration.pdf, accessed 2 March 2012).

529. *The Algiers Declaration on narrowing the knowledge gap to improve Africa's health*. June 2008. World Health Organizaton Regional Office for Africa, 2009 (http://afrolib.afro.who.int/documents/2010/En/AHM12_6_9.pdf, accessed 2 May 2012).

530. The Bamako Call to Action on Research for Health: *Strengthening research for health, development, and equity*. Bamako, Mali, 2008 (http://www.who.int/rpc/news/BAMAKOCALLTOACTIONFinalNov24.pdf, accessed 2 March 2012).

531. Commission on Health Research for Development. *Health research: essential link to equity in development*. New York: Oxford University Press, 1990.

532. WorldBank. T*he Accra Agenda for Action*. Accra, Ghana, 2008 (http://siteresources.worldbank.org/ACCRAEXT/Resources/4700790-1217425866038/AAA-4-SEPTEMBER-FINAL-16h00.pdf).

533. Nuyens Y. *No development without research: a challenge for research capacity strengthening*. Geneva, Global Forum for Health Research, 2005 (http://www.globalforumhealth.org).

534. Utzinger J, Keiser J. Schistosomiasis and soil-transmitted helminthiasis: common drugs for treatment and control. *Expert Opinion in Pharmacotherapy*, 2004, 5(2):263–285.

535. Fürst T, Keiser J, Utzinger J. Global burden of human food-borne trematodiasis: a systematic review and meta-analysis. *Lancet Infectious Diseases*, 2012, 12(3):210–221.

536. Utzinger J, A research and development agenda for the control and elimination of human helminthiases. Editorial. *PLoS Neglected Tropical Diseases*, 2012, 6(4): e1646.

537. Lustigman S et al. A research agenda for helminth diseases of humans: basic research and enabling technologies to support control and elimination of helminthiases. *PLoS Neglected Tropical Diseases*, 2012, 6(4):e1445.

538. McCarthy JS et al. A research agenda for helminth diseases of humans: diagnostics for control and elimination programmes. *PLoS Neglected Tropical Diseases*, 2012, 6(4):e1601.

539. Osei-Atweneboana MY et al. A research agenda for helminth diseases of humans: health research and capacity building in disease-endemic countries for helminthiases control. *PLoS Neglected Tropical Diseases*, 2012, 6(4):e1602.

Annex 1

The TDR disease and thematic reference groups Think Tank for Infectious Diseases of Poverty, and host countries

Reference group		Host institution and country
DRG1	Malaria	WHO country office, Cameroon
DRG2	Tuberculosis, leprosy and Buruli ulcer	WHO country office, Philippines
DRG3	Chagas disease, human African trypanosomiasis and leishmaniasis	WHO country offices, Sudan and Brazil
DRG4	Helminth infections	African Programme for Onchocerciasis Control (APOC), Burkina Faso
DRG5	Dengue and other emerging viral diseases of public health importance	WHO country office, Cuba
DRG6	Zoonoses and marginalized infectious diseases of poverty	WHO Regional Office for the Eastern Mediterranean, Egypt
TRG1	Social sciences and gender	WHO country office, Ghana
TRG2	Innovation and technology platforms for health interventions in infectious diseases of poverty	WHO country office, Thailand
TRG3	Health systems and implementation research	WHO country office, Nigeria
TRG4	Environment, agriculture and infectious diseases of poverty	WHO country office, China

Annex 2

Membership of the Disease Reference Group on Helminth Infections (DRG4)

	Name	Country	Expertise	Gender
CO-CHAIRS	Dr Sara Lustigman	USA	Molecular parasitology	F
	Dr Boakye A. Boatin	Ghana	Operational research and control measures	M
MEMBERS	Dr Rashida M. Barakat	Egypt	Parasitology	M
	Dr Guo-Jing Yang	People's Republic of China	Epidemiology	F
	Professor María-Gloria Basáñez	UK	Parasite epidemiology and modelling	F
	Dr Kwablah Awadzi	Ghana	Specialist physician	M
	Professor Banchob Sripa	Thailand	Experimental pathology	M
	Professor Warwick N. Grant	Australia	Molecular parasitology	M
	Professor Roger K. Prichard	Canada	Parasitology	M
	Dr Héctor Hugo García	Peru	Public health	M
	Professor James S. McCarthy	Australia	Tropical medicine, infectious diseases	M
	Professor Kouakou Eliézer N'Goran	Côte d'Ivoire	Parasitology, parasite ecology	M
	Dr Andrea Gazzinelli	Brazil	Social health	F

Annex 3

Composition of the TDR Think Tank

Professor Pedro Alonso, Director and Research Professor, Barcelona Centre for International Health Research (CRESIB), Barcelona, Spain

Professor Rose Leke, Head, Department of Microbiology, Immunology, Hematology and Infectious Diseases, Faculty of Medicine and Biomedical Sciences, University of Yaoundé, Yaoundé, Cameroon

Dr Joel Breman, Senior Scientific Adviser, Fogarty International Center, Division of International Epidemiology & Population Studies, National Institutes of Health, Bethesda, MD, USA

Professor Graham Brown, Foundation Director, Nossal Institute for Global Health, University of Melbourne, Carlton, Victoria, Australia

Dr Chetan Chitnis, Principal Investigator, International Centre for Genetic Engineering and Biotechnology (ICGEB), New Delhi, India

Professor Alan Cowman, Researcher, Walter and Eliza Hall Institute of Medical Research, Parkville, Victoria, Australia

Professor Abdoulaye Djimdé, Research Scientist, Chief of Laboratory, Malaria Research and Training Center (MRTC), University of Bamako, and Malian EDCTP Senior Fellow, Bamako, Mali

Dr Sócrates Herrera Valencia, Director, Caucaseco Scientific Research Center (SRC), Instituto de Inmunología del Valle, Malaria Vaccine & Drug Development Centre, Universidad del Valle, Cali, Colombia

Professor Marcelo Jacobs-Lorena, Johns Hopkins School of Public Health, Department of Molecular Microbiology and Immunology, Malaria Research Institute, Baltimore, MD, USA

Dr Ramanan Laxminarayan, Director, Center for Disease Dynamics, Economics and Policy (CDDEP), Washington, DC, USA

Professor Rosanna Peeling, Chair of Diagnostics Research, London School of Hygiene & Tropical Medicine, Department of Infectious and Tropical Diseases, Clinical Research Unit, London, England

Professor Akintunde Sowunmi, University College Hospital, Malaria Research Laboratories, Institute of Advanced Medical Research and Training (IAMRAT), Ibadan, Nigeria

Dr Sarah Volkman, Senior Research Scientist, Harvard School of Public Health, Department of Immunology and Infectious Diseases, Boston, MA, USA

Dr Tim Wells, Chief Scientific Officer, Medicines for Malaria Venture (MMV), Geneva, Switzerland

Professor Gavin Churchyard, Chief Executive Officer, Aurum Institute, Johannesburg, South Africa

Professor Charles Yu, Medical Director and Vice President for Medical Services, De La Salle Health Sciences Institute, Vice-Chancellor's Office for Mission, Cavite, Philippines

Dr Madhukar Pai, Assistant Professor, McGill University, Department of Epidemiology, Biostatistics & Occupational Health, Montreal, Quebec, Canada

Dr Ann M. Ginsberg, Senior Advisor, Global Alliance for TB Drug Development, New York, NY, USA

Dr Jintana Ngamvithayapong-Yanai, President, TB/HIV Research Foundation, Chiang Rai, Thailand

Professor Laura C. Rodrigues, Head, Department of Epidemiology and Population Health, London School of Hygiene & Tropical Medicine, London, England

Professor Martien Borgdorff, Head, Cluster Infectious Diseases, Municipal Health Service of Amsterdam and Professor of Epidemiology, University of Amsterdam, Amsterdam, Netherlands

Professor Biao Xu, Director of Tuberculosis Research Center, Professor of Epidemiology and Deputy Chair, Department of Epidemiology, School of Public Health, Fudan University, Shanghai, China

Dr Francis Adatu Engwau, Programme Manager, National Tuberculosis/Leprosy Programme, Kampala, Uganda

Dr Anthony David Harries, Senior Advisor, Director, Department of Research, London School of Hygiene & Tropical Medicine. University of London, London, England

Dr Timothy Paul Stinear, Head of Research Group NHMRC, R. Douglas Wright Research Fellow, Department of Microbiology and Immunology, University of Melbourne, Parkville, Victoria, Australia

Dr Helen Ayles, Director, ZAMBART Project, London School of Hygiene & Tropical Medicine, ZAMBART, Ridgeway Campus, University of Zambia, Lusaka, Zambia

Professor Diana Lockwood, Department of Infectious and Tropical Diseases, London School of Hygiene & Tropical Medicine, London, England

Professor Ken Stuart, President Emeritus & Founder, Seattle Biomedical Research Institute, Seattle, WA, USA

Professor Maowia M. Mukhtar, Institute of Endemic Diseases, Department of Molecular Biology, University of Khartoum, Khartoum, Sudan

Professor Bianca Zingales, Instituto de Quimica, Universidade de São Paulo, São Paulo, Brazil

Professor Marleen Boelaert, Head, Department of Public Health, Institut de Médecine Tropical, Epidemiology & Disease Control Unit, Department of Public Health, Antwerp, Belgium

Ms Marianela Castillo-Riquelme, Departamento de Economía de la Salud, DIPLAS, Subsecretaría de Salud Publica, Ministerio de Salud de Chile, Santiago, Chile

Professor Mike J. Lehane, Professor of Molecular Entomology and Parasitology, Liverpool School of Tropical Medicine, Liverpool, England

Professor Pascal Lutumba, Institut National de Recherche Bio-Médicale, Kinshasa University, Democratic Republic of the Congo

Dr Enock Matovu, Senior Lecturer, Faculty of Veterinary Medicine, Makerere University, Department of Veterinary, Parasitology and Microbiology, Kampala, Uganda

Dr David Sacks, Head, Intracellular Parasite Biology Section, National Institutes of Health, National Institute of Allergy and Infectious Diseases, Laboratory of Parasitic Diseases, Bethesda, MD, USA

Dr Sergio Alejandro Sosa-Estani, Head, Service of Epidemiology, Instituto de Efectividad Clinica y Sanitaria, Buenos Aires, Argentina

Dr Shyam Sundar, Department of Medicine, Institute of Medical Sciences, Banaras Hindu University, Varanasi, India

Professor Rick L. Tarleton, Distinguished Research Professor, Center for Tropical & Emerging Global Diseases, Coverdell Center for Biomedical Research, University of Georgia, Athens, GA, USA

Professor Alon Warburg, Professor of Vector Biology and Parasitology, The Kuvin Center for the Study of Infectious and Tropical Diseases, Faculty of Medicine, Hebrew University, Einkerem, Israel

Dr Sara Lustigman, Head, Laboratory of Molecular Parasitology, Lindsley F. Kimball Research Institute, New York Blood Center, New York, NY, USA

Dr Boakye Boatin, Noguchi Memorial Institute for Medical Research, University of Ghana, Legon, Accra, Ghana

Dr Guojing Yang, Vice Head, Department of Schistosomiasis Control, Jiangsu Institute of Parasitic Diseases, Wuxi, China

Dr Rashida M.D.R. Barakat, High Institute of Public Health, Alexandria University, Alexandria, Egypt

Dr Maria Gloria Basanez, Professor of Neglected Tropical Diseases, Department of Infectious Disease Epidemiology, Faculty of Medicine, Imperial College, London, England

Dr Kwablah Awadzi, Onchocerciasis Chemotherapy Research Centre, Hohoe Hospital, Hohoe, Ghana

Professor Banchob Sripa, Division of Experimental Pathology, Department of Pathology, Faculty of Medicine, Khon Kaen University, Khon Kaen, Thailand

Professor Warwick Grant, Head of Genetics, School of Molecular Sciences, Genetic Department, La Trobe University, Bundoora, Victoria, Australia

Professor Roger K. Prichard, Professor of Biotechnology, Institute of Parasitology, McGill University, Ste Anne de Bellevue, Quebec, Canada

Professor Hector Hugo Garcia, Department of Microbiology and Cysticercosis Unit, Instituto de Ciencias Neurologicas, Universidad Peruana Cayetano Heredia, Lima, Peru

Dr James McCarthy, Group Leader, Clinical Tropical Medicine, Queensland Institute of Medical Research, University of Queensland, Herston, Queensland, Australia

Professor Kouakou Eliezer N'Goran, Professeur de Biologie, Laboratoire de Zoologie et de Biologie Animale, Université de Cocody, Abidjan, Côte d'Ivoire

Dr Andréa Gazzinelli, School of Nursing, Federal University of Minas Gerais, Belo Horizonte, MG, Brazil

Dr Jeremy Farrar, Director, Oxford University Clinical Research Unit in Viet Nam, The Hospital for Tropical Diseases, Ho Chi Minh City, Viet Nam

Professor Maria Guzman, Head, Virology Department, Instituto de Medicina Tropical "Pedro Kouri", Havana, Cuba

Dr Natarajan Arunachalam, Senior Grade Deputy Director, Centre for Research in Medical Entomology, Indian Council of Medical Research, Madurai, India

Dr Duane Gubler, Professor, Director, Asia-Pacific Institute of Tropical Medicine and Infectious Diseases, John A Burns School of Medicine, University of Hawaii, Honolulu, HI, USA

Dr Sirirpen Kalayanarooj, Queen Sirikit National Institute of Child Health, Bangkok, Thailand

Dr Linda Lloyd, Director, Center for Research, The Institute for Palliative Medicine at San Diego Hospice, San Diego, CA, USA

Dr Lucy Chai See Lum, Associate Professor of Paediatrics, Department of Paediatrics, Faculty of Medicine, University of Malaya Medical Centre, Kuala Lumpur, Malaysia

Dr Amadou Sall, Chef de l'Unité des Arbovirus et Virus des Fièvres hémorragiques, Insitut Pasteur de Dakar, Arboviruses Unit/WHO Collaborating and Conference Centre, Dakar, Senegal

Dr Eric Martinez Torres, Instituto de Medicina Tropical Pedro Kouri, Havana, Cuba

Dr Philip J. McCall, Vector Group, Liverpool School of Tropical Medicine, Liverpool, England

Professor Derek Cummings, Assistant Professor, Department of Epidemiology, Bloomberg School of Public Health, Johns Hopkins University, Baltimore, MD, USA

Dr Hongjie Yu, Deputy Director, Professor, Office for Disease Control and Emergency Response, Chinese Center for Disease Control and Prevention, Beijing, China

Professor David Molyneux, Senior Professorial Fellow, Liverpool School of Tropical Medicine, Liverpool, England

Dr Zuhair Hallaj, Senior Consultant on Communicable Diseases, WHO Regional Office for the Eastern Mediterranean, Cairo, Egypt

Dr Gerald T. Keusch, Professor of International Health and of Medicine, Boston University, Boston, MA, USA

Dr Pilar Ramos-Jimenez, Philippine NGO Council on Population, Health and Welfare, Pasay City, Philippines

Professor Donald Peter McManus, National Health and Medical Research Council of Australia, Senior Principal Research Fellow, Head of Molecular Parasitology Laboratory, Queensland Institute of Medical Research, Brisbane, Queensland, Australia

Dr Eduardo Gotuzzo, Director, Instituto de Medicina Tropical "Alexander von Homboldt", Universidad Peruana Cayetano Heredia, Lima, Peru

Dr Kamal Kar, Chairman, CLTS Foundation, Calcutta, India

Dr Ana Sanchez, Associate Professor, Department of Community Health Sciences, Brock University, St. Catharines, Ontario, Canada

Dr Amadou Garba, Director, Réseau International Schistosomose, Environnement, Aménagement et Lutte (RISEAL), Niamey, Niger

Dr Helena Ngowi, Department of Veterinary Medicine and Public Health, Sokoine University of Agriculture, Mongoro, United Republic of Tanzania

Dr Sarah Cleaveland, Reader, Division of Ecology and Evolutionary Biology, University of Glasgow, Glasgow, Scotland

Dr Hélène Carabin, University of Oklahoma, Oklahoma Health Sciences Center, Oklahoma City, OK, USA

Professor Barbara McPake, Director and Professor, Institute for International Health and Development, Queen Margaret University, Edinburgh, Scotland

Dr Margaret Gyapong, Director, Dodowa Health Research Centre, Ghana Health Service, Dodowa, Ghana

Professor Juan Arroyo Laguna, Profesor Principal del Departamento Académico de Salud y Ciencias Sociales, FASPA-UPCH, Universidad Pruana Cayetano Heredia, Lima, Peru

Professor Sarah Atkinson, Reader, Department of Geography, University of Durham, Science Laboratories, Durham, England

Professor Rama Baru, Professor, Centre of Social Medicine and Community Health, Jawaharlal Nehru University, New Delhi, India

Professor Otto Nzapfurundi Chabikuli, Regional Technical Director, Africa Region with Family Health International (FHI360), Pretoria, South Africa

Professor Kalinga Tudor Silva, Senior Professor, Faculty of Arts, University of Peradeniya and Executive Director, International Centre for Ethnic Studies, Kandy, Sri Lanka

Professor Charles Hongoro, Research Director, Policy Analysis Unit, Human Sciences Research Council, Pretoria, South Africa

Professor Mario Mosquera-Vasquez, Associate Professor, Departamento de Comunicación Social, Universidad del Norte, Barranquilla, Colombia

Professor Chuma Jane Mumbi, Research Fellow, Kenya Medical Research Institute, Wellcome Trust Research Programme, Kilifi, Kenya Professor Helle Samuelsen, Head, Department of Anthropology, University of Copenhagen, Copenhagen, Denmark

Professor Sally Theobald, Liverpool School of Tropical Medicine, Liverpool, England

Professor Mitchell Weiss, Professor and Head of the Department of Public Health and Epidemiology Swiss Tropical Institute, Basel, Switzerland

Professor Yongyuth Yuthavong, Senior Researcher, National Centre for Genetic Engineering and Biotechnology (BIOTEC), Bangkok, Thailand

Professor Simon Croft, Professor of Parasitology, Department of Infectious and Tropical Diseases, London School of Hygiene and Tropical Medicine, London, England

Professor Rama Baru, Professor, Centre of Social Medicine and Community Health, Jawaharlal Nehru University, New Delhi, India

Professor Sanaa Botros, Manager of Training and Consultation Unit, Theodor Bilharz Research Institute, Imbaba, Giza, Egypt

Dr Mary Jane Cardosa, Director, Institute of Health and Community Medicine, University Malaysia Sarawak, Kota, Malaysia

Professor Simon Efange, Professor of Chemistry, University of Buea, Buea, Cameroon

Dr Vish Nene, Director of Biotechnology Thematic Group, International Livestock Research Institute, Nairobi, Kenya

Dr Antonio Oliveira-Dos-Santos, Medical Affairs Director, Genzyme, Rio de Janeiro, Brazil

Professor Paul Reider, Department of Chemistry, Princeton University, Princeton, NJ, USA

Dr Giorgio Roscigno, Former Chief Executive Officer, Foundation for Innovative New Diagnostics, Budé, Geneva, Switzerland

Professor Anthony So, Director, Terry Stanford Institute of Public Health Policy, Duke University, Durham, NC, USA

Professor Ming-Wei Wang, Director, The National Centre for Drug Screening, Shanghai, China

Dr Miguel Angel González-Block, Executive Director, Centre for Health Systems Research, National Institute of Public Health, Cuernavaca, Mexico

Professor Olayiwola Akinsonwon Erinosho, Executive Secretary at Health Reform Foundation of Nigeria (HERFON), Abuja, Nigeria

Dr Charles Collins, Honorary Senior Research Fellow, University of Birmingham, Birmingham, England

Dr Dyna Arhin, Associate Consultant, Public Health Action Support Team (PHAST), Faculty of Medicine, Imperial College London, England

Dr Abbas Bhuiya, Senior Social Scientist, Head, Poverty and Health Programme and Social and Behavioural Sciences Unit, Public Health Sciences Division, ICDDR,B, Mohakhali, Dhaka, Bangladesh

Dr Celia Maria de Almeida, Senior Researcher and Professor in Health Policy and Health Systems Organization, Health Administration and Planning Department, Escola Nacional de Saude Publica-ENSP/Fiocruz, Rio de Janeiro, Brazil

Professor Barun Kanjilal, Professor, Indian Institute of Health Management Research, Jaipur, India

Dr Joseph Kasonde, Executive Director, Zambia Forum for Health Research, Lusaka, Zambia

Dr Dorothée Kinde-Gazard, Minister of Health, The National AIDS Control Programme (PNLS), Cotonou, Benin

Dr Samuel Wanji, Research Foundation for Tropical Diseases and the Environment, Buea, Cameroon

Professor Anthony McMichael, Professor, National Centre for Epidemiology and Population Health, Australian National University, Canberra, ACT, Australia

Professor Xiao-Nong Zhou, Director, National Institute of Parasitic Disease, China Centers for Disease Control, Shanghai, China

Professor Corey Bradshaw, Director of Ecological Modelling, The Environment Institute and School of Earth & Environmental Sciences, University of Adelaide, Adelaide, Western Australia, Australia

Dr Stuart Gillespie, Director, RENEWAL, Coordinator, Agriculture and Health Research Platform, International Food Policy Research Institute (IFPRI), c/o UNAIDS, Geneva, Switzerland

Dr Suad M. Sulaiman, Health & Environment Adviser, Khartoum, Sudan

Professor James A. Trostle, Professor of Anthropology, Anthropology Department, Trinity College, Hartford, CT, USA

Dr Jürg Ützinger, Assistant Professor, Department of Public Health and Epidemiology, Swiss Tropical Institute, Basel, Switzerland

Professor Bruce Wilcox, Professor and Director of the Global Health Program at the University of Hawaii, Honolulu, HI, USA

Dr Guojing Yang, Assistant Professor (Principal Investigator), Dept. Schistosomiasis Control, Jiangsu Institute of Parasitic Diseases, Jiangsu Province, China

Annex 4
Distribution of the Think Tank leadership (co-Chairs)

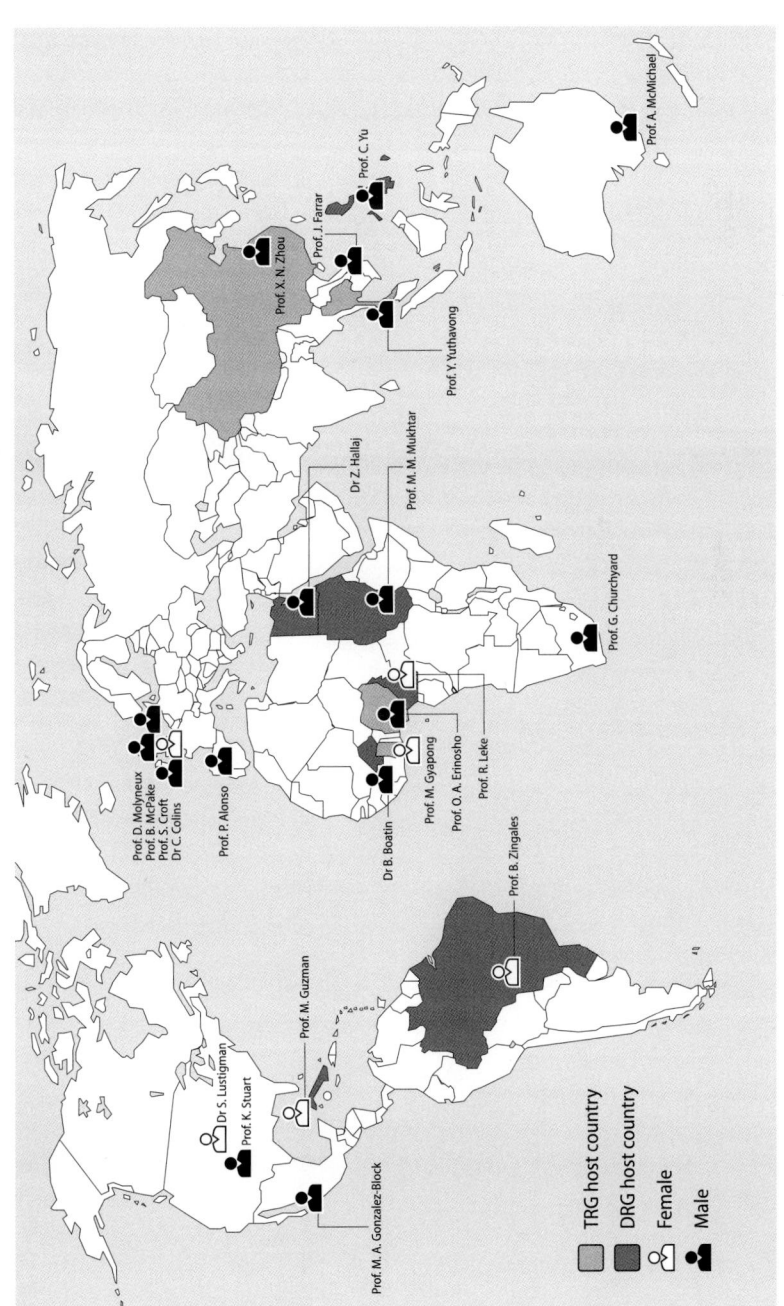

Annex 5

The top ten research priority areas for helminthiases recommended by DRG4[a]

Priority[b]	Description of priority	Ranking[c]	Helminthiasis based ranking[c,d]	
1	Optimize existing intervention tools to maximize impact (including against polyparasitism) and sustainability. The tools include pharmaceuticals, vaccines, vector control and ecohealth approaches (sanitation, clean water, improved nutrition, and education). Sustainability depends on minimizing selection for drug resistance and maintaining community support.	4.3	onchocerciasis	4.9
			LF	4.4
			STHs	4.7
			schistosomiasis	4.5
			food-borne trematodiasis	3.6
			taeniasis/cysticercosis	3.6
2	Develop novel control tools to improve impact and sustainability. The tools include pharmaceuticals, vaccines, vector control and ecohealth approaches, and how to deliver them optimally and cost effectively.	4.1	onchocerciasis	4.5
			LF	4.2
			STHs	4.3
			schistosomiasis	4.3
			food-borne trematodiasis	3.7
			taeniasis/cysticercosis	3.7
3	Improve available diagnostic tests, specifically their sensitivity, specificity, multiplex capacity, and ability to measure infection intensity and detect drug resistance. Sensitivity and specificity are mostly important to enable diagnosis of infection at low prevalence in elimination settings and to confirm cure/absence of infection.	4.1	onchocerciasis	4.9
			LF	4.2
			STHs	4.6
			schistosomiasis	4.5
			food-borne trematodiasis	3.6
			taeniasis/cysticercosis	3.3

Priority[b]	Description of priority	Ranking[c]	Helminthiasis based ranking[c,d]	
4	Standardize and validate methodologies and cost-effective protocols for diagnosis in monitoring and evaluation (M&E) settings.	3.9	onchocerciasis	4.6
			LF	4.3
			STHs	4.5
			schistosomiasis	4.3
			food-borne trematodiasis	2.7
			taeniasis/cysticercosis	3.3
5	Develop strategies incorporating delivery of multiple interventions at various levels to maximize sustainability of control programmes in general and of integrated NTD control in particular.	4.6	onchocerciasis	4.9
			LF	4.9
			STHs	4.8
			schistosomiasis	5.0
			food-borne trematodiasis	3.8
			taeniasis/cysticercosis	4.1
6	Research to develop strategies (taking gender issues into account) to increase: awareness of ill-health processes, community participation, ownership and empowerment, as well as equity in access by communities and risk groups to health services.	4.7	onchocerciasis	4.7
			LF	4.7
			STHs	4.8
			schistosomiasis	4.9
			food-borne trematodiasis	4.2
			taeniasis/cysticercosis	4.7
7	Develop and refine models to investigate the relationships between infection and morbidities to aid programmes aiming to reduce the burden of disease (elimination of public health problem). Such models need to take into account the cumulative effects of chronic disease in evaluations of disease burden, and the impact of control interventions on this burden.	3.6	onchocerciasis	4.0
			LF	3.9
			STHs	3.7
			schistosomiasis	4.0
			food-borne trematodiasis	2.8
			taeniasis/cysticercosis	3.1

Priority[b]	Description of priority	Ranking[c]	Helminthiasis based ranking[c,d]	
8	Increase the use and application of epidemiological models to aid M&E and surveillance, the design of cost-effective sampling protocols, and the monitoring of intervention efficacy including drug resistance. These models should be linked to cost-effectiveness analyses of the interventions and their alternatives.	4.0	onchocerciasis	**4.3**
			LF	**4.3**
			STHs	**4.3**
			schistosomiasis	**4.1**
			food-borne trematodiasis	3.4
			taeniasis/cysticercosis	3.4
9	Investigate how helminth parasites modulate host–parasite interactions at population and within-host levels, including impact on host immune response of concurrent infection with other helminth and non-helminth pathogens, impact of parasite control interventions on such host–parasite interactions, and how concurrent infections affect clinical outcomes and host's ability to seroconvert upon vaccination.	3.9	onchocerciasis	**4.3**
			LF	**4.4**
			STHs	**4.1**
			schistosomiasis	**4.3**
			food-borne trematodiasis	3.2
			taeniasis/cysticercosis	3.5
10	Annotate parasite genomes and transcriptomes and develop tools for parasite functional genomics in key species.	4.1	onchocerciasis	**4.8**
			LF	**4.4**
			STHs	**4.2**
			schistosomiasis	3.9
			food-borne trematodiasis	3.5
			taeniasis/cysticercosis	3.7

[a] The DRG4 collection of review papers (*496, 497, 498, 500, 507, 536, 537, 538, 539*) on 'A Research Agenda for Helminth Diseases of Humans' is available at http://www.ploscollections.org/helminths.

[b] These ten priorities are composed of the top two priorities from each of the core theme priorities that were identified (Figure 2, page 18): intervention, epidemiology and surveillance, environmental and social ecology, data and modelling, and biology. The ten priorities cannot be ranked based on importance as all of them have to be addressed similarly and in parallel – they are interconnected, and each priority will benefit from accomplishing the other priorities.

[c] Ranking of the priority research areas within the five core themes and between the six helminthiases was guided by the underlying values and criteria for ranking. Research areas were scored from 1 to 5, with 5 corresponding to the highest priority; the scores from all members of DRG4 were used to obtain the mean values.

[d] Rankings in bold indicate high priority.

Annex 6

Research landmarks and their projected impacts on the helminthiases in the short, mid and long-term periods

This was based on hypothetical time frames set for the achievement of each of the priority areas identified in time horizons of 1-5 (5), 5-15 (15) and 15-25 (25) year periods, and based on their overall impact on technological innovation, health systems and the environment.

		Potential Impacts of the top ten research priorities identified by DRG4 in:	
	Years	Area	Impact
Overall, including control of infectious diseases of poverty	5	Local National Regional	• Improved health literacy • Increased capacity building and interdisciplinary research
	15	Local National Regional	• Much improved health literacy and education, integrated health intervention for polyparasitism, multi- and interdisciplinary research • Potential elimination of onchocerciasis/LF as a public health problem in many foci and elimination of infection in some foci
	25	Local National Regional	• Equity in health literacy, improved universal access to interventions • Fully Integrated health interventions • Major reduction of disease burden due to helminthiases
Technological innovations	5	Local	• Mobile phone and PDA reporting systems (mapping GIS and surveillance)
		National Regional	• Optimized drug combinations and treatment regimens • Refined models for infection and morbidities relationships • Improved diagnostic tests (sensitivity, specificity) for low intensity infections • Biomarkers for drug resistance
	15	Local	• Implementation of the use of novel diagnostics for low intensity infections • Markers of drug resistance improve operational MDA strategies
		National	• Tools for parasite functional genomics in key species • Accurate burden of disease/ infection are defined
		Regional	• Drugs, vaccines, and vector control tools from bio-technology • Partnerships produce drugs, vaccines and biomarker assays

	Years	Area	Impact
Potential Impacts of the top ten research priorities identified by DRG4 in: *(continued)*			
Technological innovations	25	Local National Regional	• Disease-endemic countries produce own drugs, vaccines, biomarkers and vector control tools • Equity in health technology in disease endemic countries
Health systems	5	Local	• Increased community participation, ownership and empowerment • New improved community-directed interventions
	5	National Regional	• Standardized and validated methodologies and protocols for diagnosis in M&E settings • Epidemiological models to aid M&E and surveillance are developed • Impact of intervention on the host immune response can be taken into consideration for MDA operational strategies
	15	Local National Regional	• Maximized commitment to sustainability of control programmes in general and to integrated NTD control in particular • Models for co-infection and models for the impact of climate change on helminth infections support health systems decisions
	25	Local	• Equity in access by communities and risk groups to health services, and gender issues considered
		National Regional	• Integrated NTD control fully in place
Environmental	5	Local	• Implementation of sanitation (community led total sanitation), including availability of potable water
		National	• Models for the impact of climate change on helminth infections are developed
		Regional	• Vaccines against zoonotic reservoirs (e.g. pigs, bovines) • Better and more complex early warning systems, including disaster preparedness for more extreme weather
	25	Local National Regional	• Sanitation for all in disease endemic countries, with markedly improved water management